Married to Alzheimer's

Married to Alzheimer's

A life less ordinary with Tony Booth

Steph Booth

RIDER

LONDON • SYDNEY • AUCKLAND • JOHANNESBURG

3 5 7 9 10 8 6 4 2

Rider, an imprint of Ebury Publishing,
20 Vauxhall Bridge Road,
London SW1V 2SA

Rider is part of the Penguin Random House group of companies
whose addresses can be found at global.penguinrandomhouse.com

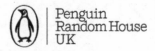

| Penguin
Random House
UK

First published by Rider in 2019

www.penguin.co.uk

A CIP catalogue record for this book is available from the British Library

HB ISBN 9781846045752
TPB ISBN 9781846045769

Typeset in 11.75/17.5 pt Garamond MT Pro
by Integra Software Services Pvt. Ltd, Pondicherry

Printed and bound in Great Britain by Clays Ltd, Elcograf S.p.A.

Penguin Random House is committed to a sustainable future for
our business, our readers and our planet. This book is made
from Forest Stewardship Council® certified paper.

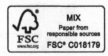

This book is a work of non-fiction based on the experiences and recollec-
tions of Steph Booth. In some cases names of people and sequences of the
detail of events have been changed to protect the privacy of others.

for Tony

Contents

He was my North, my South, my East and West,
My working week and my Sunday rest,
My noon, my midnight, my talk, my song;
I thought that love would last for ever: I was wrong.

W.H. Auden, 'Funeral Blues'

Introduction

This is the story of my life with the actor and campaigner Tony Booth, and how we coped with his Alzheimer's. It is the truth of our marriage and the impact dementia had on us as a couple and the life we had together. This book, *Married to Alzheimer's*, has developed from the columns I wrote for the *Irish Times* about living with Tony's Alzheimer's, which in turn came out of a discussion Tony and I had about his involvement in the National Pensioners Convention (NPC). When Tony and I discussed going public about his illness he was initially uncertain. He was embarrassed to have Alzheimer's, but after some reflection he told me I should write the pieces, saying, 'If I'm ashamed, what about those other poor buggers? Let's get it out in the open, it's about time.' It was obviously personally difficult for him, but he saw it as the next logical step in his campaign for pensioner rights. One of the ironies of all this was that Tony never accepted he had dementia. He would accept he had Alzheimer's, it was a disease that showed up on his brain scan, but not dementia.

He refused to be labelled 'demented' with all those negative connotations.

Tony was always an active political campaigner and his fame as an actor gave him a voice and a national platform which he was never reticent about using. The framing of older people as a drain on public finances and resources would infuriate him and once his son-in-law became the Prime Minister, Tony had even more opportunity to make his opinions known. He seized on every chance to lecture Tony Blair about the inadequacy of UK provision for the elderly. Poor man. No wonder he was so often busy when we stayed at Number 10.

It was while we were living in Ireland that Tony was first diagnosed with Alzheimer's. It was only a tentative diagnosis and as nothing much changed in our day-to-day lives, it was easy enough to push it to the back of my mind as something that might or might not get worse. This was still in the early years of our marriage and our life was happy. Looking back, I can see we were incredibly lucky to have had that time in Ireland together. Away from the stresses and strains of life back in England, we were able to focus on each other, learning how to live together and establishing the give and take of a loving if tempestuous relationship. In that situation, who wants to think about the possibility of what life might eventually have in store? Certainly not me, and Tony had point-blank refused to accept he might be in the early stages of dementia. The head-in-the-sand strategy suited us both very well.

It was a couple of years after our return to England that the prognosis that had existed on the fringes of our lives suddenly demanded centre stage. That's when everything changed. With the benefit of hindsight, I realise I was embarrassed and wondered how long we might be able to keep Tony's dementia a secret. How would I cope with the reactions of other people? I was not quite the hero I had imagined or hoped I would be, but despite this wobble I did somehow manage to overcome these feelings. At least most of the time.

Dementia is a cruel disease. It destroys an individual's personality bit by agonising bit and the misery of seeing that happen is unspeakable. It is not a disease like cancer or heart failure, where research and the medical professions can offer time lines, medical support and – in the case of cancer – the hope of remission. Dementia is unique to the person who has it and does not fit neatly into medical or research boxes. All we can do is wait and watch to see what happens next.

I went through some really tough times looking after Tony. The mood swings, the incessant repetition of the same question or statement. The hardest time was when Tony knew something was wrong with him but he couldn't work out what it was. Sometimes his roaring frustration would fill the whole day and he would be threatening me with 'his lawyers', meaning his daughters Cherie and Lyndsey. I would sometimes respond with threats of my own – specifically that if he didn't stop behaving in this way he would have to go to live in a home. Usually, I would take the dogs for a long walk to escape from him and manage my own anger, exhaustion and desire to walk out on him for ever. For some reason I didn't ever walk out, maybe because I would eventually manage to get some sleep, which would always help.

Caring for Tony was always an up-and-down experience, and it was hard to keep up. He was restless at nights and I found sleep deprivation hard to cope with. Changing his medication helped, but as a result he became much more passive. Perversely, I was heartbroken. Where had my Tony gone? As well as making sure he didn't become irritable, I now had to be alert to his tiredness, particularly as his physical health was deteriorating. Having smoked since he was eleven years old, he was now suffering from heart failure. This was yet another layer of concern for me.

One of the hardest things to accept – and I have yet to come to terms with it – is how little there is in the way of meaningful, long-term support for those suffering from Alzheimer's and for the people who care for them. Leaving the doctor's office after being told the results of Tony's brain scan was one of the loneliest and most unnerving moments of my life. What was I supposed to do? Where was the information and advice? I didn't even know if Alzheimer's was a psychological or a physical illness. Thank goodness for Google as the information really wasn't forthcoming from anywhere else.

This was more than ten years ago and sadly I don't see that the situation has particularly improved. Information is power and even the most basic facts would enable carers to get to grips and cope with what might happen as dementia progresses. While a great deal of money is spent on research, too little is put into providing essential information for carers, including letting them know how to access social service care and what benefits they might be entitled to.

Once I had made the decision to look after Tony myself – that he was not going into a care home – it was a case of muddling through. As his illness progressed, Tony became more and more dependent on me, which was exhausting and often frustrating; but having him at home meant I also got all the good as well as the bad. The times when he was lucid and chatty were a joy, and I could almost pretend things were fine. As his wife and carer, I was determined that we were going to continue to have as normal a life as possible, with the same routines, the same expectations of holidays and days out, keeping up with friends, pottering around at home and in the garden. Tony and I continued to have some really good holidays; he loved Paris and we went there quite often as one of my sons lived there. Heart failure meaning that he could no longer fly, he once persuaded me to drive all the way from West Yorkshire to south of Carcassonne in Languedoc. He was a history buff and particularly interested in the Cathars and their castles, which were always found on the top of cliffs. However, once we were there and he saw how steep the mountains were, I was the one despatched to climb them, take photographs of the castles and then show him what I had seen. What a dutiful wife I was!

I learned quickly that it is not only the carer who has to adapt. Family and friends are also captured by the dementia bubble. Tony started to retreat into his own world and while he could still recognise us, he did not always communicate effectively. He had an often distant and sometimes fraught relationship with his daughters and their absence from his life made connections with them even more difficult. It was excruciating and I felt for them when he eventually did not know who they were, and they were clearly taken aback, even hurt by this failure. We inevitably reached a point in his decline where he didn't or couldn't make the effort to recognise most people, although I was sometimes surprised by who he did remember. Gale, the mother of his daughters Cherie and Lyndsey, was one. They were tied by their shared past and would chat and reminisce contentedly about family members. They never ran out of things to say to each other, happily revisiting the same stories.

Up until a few weeks before Tony died, he was still up and about, managing to get down the stairs to his armchair and be part of the household. But one morning it all changed. He woke up and couldn't get out of bed. He had simply run out of strength. A hospital bed was brought in and we now had help from the district nurses. He stopped eating and I knew then that we were at the beginning of the end. I wanted to make sure that every one of his family and friends who wanted to see him before he died was able to do so. This was testing for me as what I really wanted to do was close the door on the world and keep this last precious time with Tony for myself. He had visitors daily and he was pleased to see people, but I was a firm gatekeeper, watching and making sure he wasn't becoming too tired. Although he slept a lot, the nights were restless and the baby alarm kept me running up and down the stairs to settle him.

It was during one of our last conversations that Tony made me promise to finish writing this book, which I had begun a few months before he died. He was very proud of me, talking about 'my wife the writer'. He believed it was important to tell people what living with Alzheimer's was really like for the carer. Tony wanted this book to be the voice of the ordinary person, the experience from the grassroots telling it like it really is. He would encourage, nag and persuade me to keep writing even when I found it too emotionally challenging and too tiring to continue.

I understand our solution cannot for so many reasons be the right one for everyone who has a relative with dementia. Whatever your choice, there will always be guilt, sadness, loss and grief. There is no escape from that fact it is something we have to learn to live with. If this is your situation, the one thing I will say categorically is that the right and best solution is the one that works for you. It really is that simple.

I want this book to show others going through a similar experience that they are not alone, that we are all just human beings doing our best, in the only way we know how – and that is absolutely fine. Whatever your situation, I hope you will find something in this book that will help you to know there are so many more of us out there on the same journey. Mine is just one story.

1.

The beginning

Nothing in my life previously could possibly have prepared me for Tony Booth. We met in 1996, on a glorious August evening at a mutual friend's garden party. It was not a meeting of minds, despite Tony telling me later that he had been watching me from a window and later claiming it was, for him at least, love at first sight – although he had a strange way of demonstrating it. Making his entrance into the garden, he came over to talk to me and asked during our conversation if I had any holiday plans. I told him I was about to take my children camping in France. He was horrified that, as a woman alone, I would even contemplate such a thing and felt he should give me the benefit of his opinion about the foolhardiness of this venture. Fortunately, someone else came over to talk to him and I was able to excuse myself and wander away, spending the rest of the evening chatting to other people. I was taken aback by Tony's rudeness. What on earth had my holiday choices got to do with him? I was later to learn Tony had never forgiven the French for the

Norman invasion and, as such, they were never to be trusted, particularly on their own territory. The fact I was going to Brittany rather than Normandy appeared to be an irrelevant fact, even though the Bretons were, by all accounts, a different quality of people. That conversation was the start of it all, the clash of two opinionated, strong-willed people. Looking back, I'm not sure how we made it – but we did and I miss him so very much.

When Tony and I met, he was going through a divorce from his then wife, Nancy Jaeger, whom he had married perhaps a little too quickly after the death of his wife Pat Phoenix. He couldn't bear to be alone. I had also been in an unhappy marriage and, having been divorced for a few years, I wanted to put all that unhappiness behind me when I moved from Devon to West Yorkshire. I had been offered a funded master's degree at the University of Bradford to research gender and civil society. This was an opportunity too good to pass up and due to the somewhat surprising but gratefully accepted generosity of the NatWest bank, I was able to take out a mortgage on a tiny, back-to-back terrace house in Hebden Bridge. The town was on a direct rail link to Bradford and in 1995, when I bought it, housing was still affordable there. It had not become the upmarket, somewhat twee place of current legend. It was an excellent and positive opportunity for a new start for me and my two youngest sons, Sam and Will.

Soon after returning from France I bumped into Tony and this time he was the charming, solicitous chap that only he could be, expressing huge interest in my holiday. He asked me out for lunch and I agreed. It was only later he told me he was suffering from ill health and eating was problematic for him. We really enjoyed ourselves, talking non-stop for hours, but even then we disagreed (mildly) on a few issues. On reflection, we seemed to move quickly from lunch to seeing a lot of each other, discovering a shared enthusiasm for films, books and politics. Tony's conviction and belief in socialism and the Labour Party were embedded in his DNA. Coming from his background of Liverpool Irish Catholicism, he couldn't be anything else. My family are Manchester Irish Catholics and while this could and did create issues between us on the footballing front, it also meant we had a lot in common, including our politics. Tony often spoke about his grandfather, Robert Thompson, campaigning in the 1945 general election; I recall my grandmother telling me of her delight as a working-class woman who voted Labour in the same election, knowing they were going to win. For so many people at that time Labour really was the bright new dawn. Like Robert Thompson, she had high hopes for a practical socialist future. Thank goodness neither of them were alive for the Thatcher government.

Although Tony had campaigned and worked for the Labour Party for decades – he had been friends with Harold Wilson, Barbara Castle, Michael Foot and Tony Benn – I only became active in Labour politics when Margaret Thatcher's government was elected. Both Tony and I supported the

1984–5 miners' strike, both working and hoping for a Labour government, yet oblivious to each other's existence. I was a little minnow busying away in the shallows of leafleting and door knocking, while he and his wife Pat Phoenix were stars of the movement. It's funny how life can turn out.

Of course, our courtship was overshadowed by the upcoming general election of May 1997; it was an exciting time politically and it was during the early months of 1997 that I met Tony's eldest daughter, Cherie, for the first time. It was at an event in Liverpool and she was accompanied by the ever impressive Fiona Millar, who was her advisor. Cherie was keen to know the details of my relationship with her dad and we managed to find time for a quick gossip before she moved on to the next event.

Interest in Tony and, by default, me increased as the election approached and anything and anyone remotely connected to Tony's daughter Cherie and her husband, Tony Blair, became fair game as far as the press were concerned. I don't recall what my Tony was filming at the time, but he was being interviewed on the set by a reporter who, of course, wanted to talk about the Blairs as well as about his divorce from Nancy, all of which he handled with his usual aplomb. Despite his reputation as a loose cannon – and he could be one – before any interview, Tony would usually think carefully about the points he wanted to make. (Some of those so-called loose cannon moments were entirely deliberate.) However, on this occasion the reporter suddenly switched her attention to me and asked, 'Are you and Tony planning to have a baby?'

'Mind your own business,' was my immediate and surprised response.

'Oh, but it is my business. Our readers have a right to know.'

Really? Tony was a well-known figure and like all actors he relied on press interest to keep himself in the public eye. I was not a public figure, but I was and am governed by basic courtesy and felt the need to make a response, so I simply said, 'That's not something we've discussed.' Silly me. I would never make such a basic mistake now – an open-ended remark, ripe for interpretation in whatever way the reporter chose. And, to be perfectly honest, nor would I now feel the need to respond to such an intrusive question.

While all this was going on around us, Tony and I decided to move in together, which meant learning how to live with each other. No mean feat for either of us. I honestly think, particularly in the beginning, it was because Tony was still working fairly regularly and would quite often be away that we both had the space we needed. He loved being surrounded by people; he hoovered up that energy and thrived on it. While I love being around people, I on the other hand need time and space to be alone. I am happy in my own company and this was one of the reasons a garden became an essential component of our relationship, as it provided me with an accessible bolt hole. Being out there gave me the peace I wanted, but it was also a space where we could entertain. Having friends round for a meal was something we were good at as a couple and we quickly established a great dynamic. I love to cook and Tony was an excellent master of ceremonies, keeping the conversation and laughter flowing. The atmosphere could sometimes loosen the tongues of even the most shy.

One of our closest friends, John, is a GP and a quiet sort of chap, but one night he surprised everyone with a story about a pineapple, a rectum and a painful few hours in A&E for one individual. Unsurprisingly, this was a tale that Tony never forgot and he would always preface its retelling with the words, 'My mate John, who is a doctor ...' Sometimes we were almost too good at making our friends feel at home and I remember when it got particularly late one evening and Tony disappeared, only to reappear a few minutes later in his pyjamas, holding his toothbrush. Fortunately, this was taken in good humour by our guests, with everyone seeing it for the joke it was. It seemed then that we had so much to live for, with so many plans for the future, but gradually – like so much else – these lively, sociable suppers became a thing of memory.

It is in the garden where I think about Tony the most. I sit or wander around, looking at our plants and remembering when and where we bought them. Tony never objected to spending money on the garden. It was a kind of quid pro quo arrangement on expenses: I planted and he smoked. When he was a boy, Tony lived with his family in a terraced house in

Liverpool. The house had a tiny front garden and to please his mother, Vera, Tony would cadge seeds and cuttings from the local park keeper, which he would try to grow in their small plot. I don't know if it is still there, but he always claimed a rose that climbed up the front of the house was a testament to his green-fingered endeavours.

There is a strong, almost primal energy in many of us that wants to create a garden even in the most unpromising of sites. I remember my grandmother, who also lived in a terraced house, trying to create a garden in her backyard. She was not very successful as she thought a few inches of soil on top of the flags would be sufficient for plants to put down roots. She was far better at persuading the local birds to gather on her outside windowsill to eat toast crumbs she'd made especially for them at breakfast time. They would tap on the window with their beaks if they thought she wasn't supplying them quickly enough.

I've probably inherited my own love of garden birds from my grandmother, as I've always fed them and encouraged them into our garden. Tony would spend ages watching them from the window as they took full advantage of the various avian fast-food centres (aka bird feeders) out there. It makes me think of the cafe in Hathersage where our friends Brian and Betty would take us whenever we visited them in Derbyshire. It's a pleasant place, but the real highlight is the lovely bird tables near the stream: a magnificent selection of birds come to these well-stocked tables. As dementia caused Tony's world to shrink, it was good to see he could still connect with, and take pleasure in, watching beautiful, living things. His imagination had not completely shut down.

I read a *Guardian* article online recently about research that has shown how gardens can specifically improve the health of people with dementia by raising spirits, relieving stress and providing an activity to share with family and friends. I certainly found this to be true for Tony, which is why in the late winter/early spring of 2017 I decided on a complete redesign of our garden. Our house is situated on the side of a valley, so the garden is steep and terraced, which was always going to be an issue for Tony as he became more unsteady on his feet. A gently sloping, meandering path was created, the plan being to enable Tony to enjoy the garden the following summer. However, it rains a lot in West Yorkshire in February. With the garden soon starting to resemble a First World War trench, I began to despair at the decision I had made. So did the cats, who would occupy the window sill, staring out at the horror of it all. That spring, despite or perhaps because of the chaos in the garden, the frogs went into overdrive on the spawning front. With frog spawn bubbling over the sides of the pond, it looked like an amphibian orgy had taken place. Tony was deeply impressed by their stamina.

*

The garden has always given me a sense of peace whenever I find life a little tough. These days, I understand Churchill's 'black dog' better than ever, as he occasionally sits on my shoulder too. The miseries will last three days, with the second being the toughest, and then they go away. I understand myself well enough to hang on in there, in the knowledge that these feelings are the inevitable, long-term fallout from my troubled childhood. I am the oldest of five children, all born over an eight-year period, so even as a little girl I was expected to relieve my mother of some of the pressure of maternal duties.

I never had an easy relationship with my mother. She blamed me, as she repeatedly made clear, for having to marry my father. They were married in June 1954 and I was born in January 1955. With so many children – they kept going until they had a son – and my father only ever working in poorly paid jobs, life was tough. We rarely had new clothes and our wardrobe was made up of other kids' cast-offs, or the things my mother stitched and knitted. She was not very good at needlework and I still recall, with a sense of squirming humiliation, being the butt of cruel comments in the school playground. I dreaded play-time, but I loved school. I was smart and realised that, if I worked really hard, this would be my way to achieve success – a passage to a better life. At primary school my aim was to pass the eleven-plus entrance exam to the local grammar school, and I did.

I told Tony some things about my childhood, but not everything – I haven't ever told anyone the full story. Our upbringing shapes and defines us and no matter how well I cope, there are still a few things likely to put me in meltdown. Understanding my anxieties, Tony was always very protective towards me in any situation where he thought I might feel threatened. He was not the world's most sensitive or tactful man, but he understood this much. If I leaned into him, he would automatically kiss my forehead, a deeply comforting action, something he did almost without thinking. Sometimes he would look at me and say, 'You need a hug.' It was not a question but a statement of fact, and I would just have to nod to be enveloped in his strong, caring arms. It is impossible to describe the absolute relief that can come from a simple action.

On the other hand, Tony could be an absolute egotistical monster when things weren't going his way. If I had a pound for every time he said he was leaving, I would be a wealthy woman. My goodness, did he ever love a dramatic – even histrionic – moment. When I first encountered this behaviour I was completely taken aback. How on earth was I supposed to deal with that? However, I got used to it and when he kicked off I would offer to go and get his bag for him, beating him to his punch line, 'That's it, I'm leaving.'

What is it with men and their 'threatening to leave' dramas? I remember when Will, my youngest son, was about twelve and suspended from school after he and his friend Rob hid their science teacher's lab keys. Our friend Brian, who was the deputy head at the school, telephoned to say Will was on his way home. After a heated debate with my son, who could not understand why I was not being more supportive, he announced he was leaving. Dragging his loaded bag downstairs, he asked me to take him to the station. I refused, so he dragged his bag back upstairs and slammed shut his bedroom door, not to reappear until hunger forced him out. Among our family and friends Brian is a legend who is always introduced as the man who suspended Will.

Given his dramatic tendencies, Tony's marriage proposal in the autumn of 1997 was surprisingly low-key, so much so that I didn't actually hear what he was saying. In fact I was half asleep because we were in the car and Tony was driving. He was a terrible driver, forever taking his hands off the wheel when he was talking and waving his hands about to emphasise various points. I always tried to doze in this situation, so I didn't have to watch and panic as death approached. Aware he had said something important, I replied, 'I'm sorry, I didn't quite catch that.' Sighing heavily, he repeated himself, turning up the volume. I heard him that time, but I didn't know what to say. My lack of an immediate or positive response started to make him cross that the moment had been ruined. I asked him to stop the car so we could get out. Then I walked round the car, put my arms around him, said yes – and that was that.

Initially, we planned to marry in a local registry office and even went as far as setting a date, but then we learned quickly that our plans had been leaked to the newspapers, so we cancelled the venue. We turned to Cherie for advice. She is a formidable organiser who soon had everything sorted. And so we were married in Liverpool at the Devonshire House Hotel. We then went on to St Francis de Sales Church in Walton, where Tony's cousin John was the priest, for a blessing. For me, it was a nerve-shredding moment as we turned the corner and saw the press scrum waiting for us at the church. Cherie and Tony had already arrived, travelling from the Labour Party Conference in Blackpool with the media in hot pursuit, as they were aware of our plans. Noticing my rising panic, our driver said, 'OK, lots of deep breaths, keep your knees together when you get out of the car, keep looking straight ahead and just go for it.' I'm certain there were far more important things going on in the world that day than our wedding, but you wouldn't have thought so. But in the end it couldn't have gone more smoothly. It was the perfect wedding and a lot of people put a great deal of effort into making it happen. I've been Mrs Booth since 2 October 1998.

We didn't plan to have a honeymoon, we were hardly love's young dream; and besides which, Tony was busy working and I was researching and writing my doctorate. However, one afternoon I answered a telephone call from Tony's agent, John Markham, who asked if we would like to go to Jamaica. I knew there would be a catch and there was. As the saying goes, 'There ain't no such thing as a free lunch.' The trip was offered by *Hello* magazine as they wanted a large, several-page photographic feature of Tony and me on honeymoon. I immediately said no. John was surprised, thinking I would jump at the opportunity of a free holiday in the Caribbean, but I was adamant I didn't want anything to do with it. Poor man, he thought it would be a nice surprise for me. Later that day he phoned Tony, who was definitely up for a holiday and positive publicity. I was harassed by the pair of them into going, but I was still uncertain. As things turned out, I shouldn't have been so churlish. The *Hello* article took only a couple of days out of the two weeks we spent there. The rest of the time Tony and I pottered about, reading, sunbathing and snoozing.

One of the things I really enjoyed on the holiday was going scuba diving for the first time. The diving was organised by the hotel and the only qualification was to be able to swim a width of the hotel pool under water. Easy peasy. It was a fantastic experience, sitting at the bottom of the Caribbean Sea with the most beautiful and colourful shoals of fish swimming past, around my outstretched arms. Tony stayed on the boat, waiting for me. With his damaged skin, badly burnt in a house fire, he was not a happy swimmer, but he wanted to enjoy the experience vicariously and see me come up safely.

I went down a second time a few days later, but we had to come up sooner than anticipated as sharks were circling and there was no time to waste. Much to my amusement, Tony was soaking wet when I got back on the boat. There had been a cloud burst while we were diving. He was not pleased. In fact, he wanted to talk about just how wet he was much more than he wanted to reflect on the possibility of his wife being eaten alive by sharks. So sensitive and empathetic, my husband.

In the dentist's waiting room a few months after our Jamaica trip, I was idly flicking through a stack of *Hello* magazines. Of course, I had seen the article when it was published, but I had not thought about it being so widely available in public places months after publication. When I saw it again in the dentist of all places, I was embarrassed to say the least. Furtively looking round to make sure no one was watching, I put the magazine back at the bottom of the pile so no one else could find it. Just as I was about to relax, one of the other waiting patients laughed and said, 'It's OK, Steph, I've already read it.' She had seen my name. Thank goodness I'd refused all requests to have my photograph taken in my swimsuit. Imagine the mortification.

Tony and I travelled a lot, mainly holidays on the Continent, but in the early days of our marriage I was still working on my doctorate when I was asked to present an academic paper in New York. I had come a long way from that little girl who just wanted to pass her eleven-plus exam. The university paid my expenses, which was very useful. Tony came with me because he wanted to go on a jolly and also because his two daughters with Julie Allan, Jenia and Bronwen, were living in New York at the time and it was a good opportunity to see them. What a brilliant city, we both loved it. We stayed at the Gramercy Park Hotel. As Tony so succinctly put it, if it was good enough for Humphrey Bogart and James Cagney then it had to be good enough for us. He had also managed to wangle a flight upgrade by mentioning to the people at check-in that his eldest daughter, whose address happened to be 10 Downing Street, was one of the emergency contacts in his passport. It worked on the flight home, too.

We arrived in New York in the late afternoon, with just enough time for a quick nap before the evening session of a socialist conference where Noam Chomsky was to be a key speaker. A friend of ours knew somebody who lived in New York, who had invited us to the event as Tony's politics were well known and he thought we might be interested. As guests, Tony and I were given the best seats in the house, in the middle of the front row.

Unfortunately, whilst it was early evening in New York, my body clock was still set to the Greenwich meridian and believed it was time for bed. I find some of Chomsky's work quite interesting, but his lecture style is not the liveliest. I put my head on Tony's shoulder to rest my eyes for a few moments and the inevitable happened. I didn't just fall asleep, I fell so deeply asleep to the point where I was dribbling down

Tony's shoulder. He tried to wake me several times, but I was a hopeless case. I hoped Mr Chomsky hadn't noticed me, but at the end of the evening when Tony and I were introduced to him, he remarked on how tired I must be. Blazing, shamed cheeks for me. When everyone went home, Tony and I were somewhat surprised as we were used to Labour Party meetings and conferences, where some of the best discussion takes place in pubs and bars after the main event. The Americans obviously take socialism far more seriously than we do. Though, to be honest, on this occasion we were relieved to get to our bed.

While we were in New York, one of Tony's key missions was to visit Katz's Deli for a pastrami on rye. We arrived at lunchtime and were shown to a table. I didn't realise the deli was as famous for its obstreperous staff as for its food. We had an elderly waitress who, for whatever reason, seemed to find Tony and I quite tiresome. When we finished lunch, Tony disappeared to the washroom and I headed for the cash register. While I was waiting to pay our bill, I spotted Tony and waved to him. Focused on reaching me, he failed to spot the elderly waitress who appeared as if out of nowhere as he passed our table. She rugby tackled him, almost bringing him to the floor. Horrified, I shouted, 'Oh my God, that woman is attacking my husband!' With other diners turning to look and Tony trying to push the waitress off him, a more senior member of staff tried to calm the situation and explained the waitress thought Tony was trying to leave without paying, or more importantly leave without giving her a tip. I can think of more appropriate ways in which she might have dealt with the situation, but I settled up promptly and we left in search of a coffee house where we could recover our wits and dignity.

Sadly, I didn't manage to complete my doctorate in the end. Tony was writing his autobiography, *What's Left?*, in 2001 and little by little I was pulled into writing it for him as I turned his stream-of-consciousness notes into something more readable and non-libellous. After explaining my situation to the University of Salford, I was assured that when I was ready I would be able pick up the funding again and complete my research. When I made enquiries recently about doing so, I found that sadly it was no longer the case. I was naturally disappointed as I would really have liked to finish it, particularly now I have more time. Cultural identity and civil society are still as relevant now as they were a few years ago, but I suppose, as with many other things, academic fashions change.

While Tony was able to go to New York and academic conferences with me, I attended parties and film and television events with him. Tony played Lord Antonio in the film *Revengers Tragedy*. It was released in the UK at the beginning of 2003, with a premiere in Liverpool. At the drinks party afterwards, a young woman came up to talk to Tony and me. Well, just Tony really. She gradually interposed herself between us until I was left looking at her back. Not pleased, I moved around and, touching Tony's arm, asked him to go and get me a drink. A glass of dry white wine would be perfect. This left me alone with a woman who was clearly only willing to make small talk with me until Tony came back.

'Are you an actor?' she asked.

'No.'

'Well, do you work in the business?'

'No.'

Looking me up and down in a not very kind fashion, she then asked, 'So what are you doing with Tony Booth?'

Smiling, I replied, 'Because he's a really good fuck and he happens to be my husband.' I have no idea what possessed me, but her face was adequate revenge for her rudeness. She was stunned.

As Tony approached with my wine, he read the situation perfectly. 'I see you've met my lady wife,' he said, handing me the glass and then, taking my elbow, he guided me away whilst telling the young woman we really had to mingle. 'Dear God, woman, I really can't take you anywhere!' he said as he struggled not to laugh.

We all have those moments of extraordinary, out-of-character behaviour we remember for years and this is one of those moments for me. I still can't make up my mind if I should be proud or ashamed of it.

*

Apart from the occasional glamorous moments, the early years of our marriage were just like those in any relationship. Settling down together, we rowed and fought, loved and laughed, were happy and sometimes sad, and generally faced up to the fact that if the relationship is worth anything then so is trying harder when the going gets tough. Easy to say, but not always that easy to carry through when running away sometimes seems by far the easiest option.

One of the things I initially struggled to cope with was the extent of Tony's dope smoking. I was used to people smoking dope occasionally, but when I first met Tony, he was smoking every night and at some point during the day he would go through his ritual of preparation for the evening indulgence, when he would chain-smoke his joints. I don't know the effect this level of dope has on other people, but it certainly wasn't always pleasant being around Tony. Quite often he would just pass out in his chair, but this was when I first knew him and he was under a lot of stress. Things did improve the longer we were together, as he cut back his consumption and somehow, as we always seemed to do, we muddled through. Looking back, I can see it is a good thing none of us knows what the future might bring. We would be bailing out if we knew some of the choices we would have to make and the issues we would have to face. Thank goodness I was blissfully unaware of the damage Tony's drug use was going to do to his brain and the effect that would have on both our lives.

One of my favourite recording artists is Tracy Chapman, and her song with the lines 'If you knew that you would die today...would you change?' has always hit me hard, especially since Tony died. It is such a poignant, bittersweet question. I don't know the answer, but I do know I would have missed out on having rose petals scattered on my bed in the early days when my husband was madly in love with me. We wouldn't have got lost in Thirsk (the Bermuda Triangle of North Yorkshire) the first time we went away together, but then, once we'd escaped, found a really good hotel. I would not have had so much life and love and I would not have had the funny, everyday memories that sustain me now as I struggle to come to terms with my new normal. His Alzheimer's meant I was losing Tony over a long period of time and I was never going to get him back, but from those early days we had fashioned an instinctive, warts-and-all understanding of one another and that was the bedrock of our relationship. A marriage that included not just us, but, as in so many other modern marriages, children from other relationships and all the complexities and emotional baggage that brings with it.

2.

The family

T ony and I have twelve children between us. Well, I know I definitely have four sons, but with Tony it's a little more complicated. He has eight daughters that I know of. When I first met him there were seven, until Lucy, who had been living in Australia and whom none of us knew about, made it eight. It was a minor concern before Tony's funeral about what to do if any more women turned up at the church claiming to be either unknown offspring or unknown partners. Given his early, rackety lifestyle, this was entirely possible. I decided dignity and graciousness would be the only proper ways to handle it. As far as I'm aware, no one we weren't expecting turned up, so best behaviour wasn't called for on the matter. But I'm pretty cool about these things anyway. I always took the attitude that what happened before he met me, in terms of his relationships, was exactly that: *ante*-Steph.

It is in other areas of my life that I can sometimes be overwhelmed. The past can be difficult to cope with at times and as a consequence I have always lived with an underlying sense of anxiety and fear. As I have got older, I can understand my desperate history of broken relationships is very much the legacy of a dysfunctional childhood driven and shaped by violent and unloving parents. My father was a particularly violent, sadistic and abusive man, a crime my mother colluded in with her unquestioning acceptance of his behaviour. I remember years later confronting her about it. Why did she not protect me? She simply shrugged her shoulders and asked what I had expected her to do. The pain of that response remains with me still. Now, with greater public awareness and less shame, I understand how manipulative all abusers are, and my father was no different, but that makes it no less difficult to deal with when the shadows creep up behind me.

Surviving such a childhood is one thing, but knowing how to make adult relationships work is quite another. If you don't understand what it means to give and take, love and work hard, compromising where necessary, if you don't understand the fundamentals, then making relationships work is tough. What is 'normal' apart from obviously not behaving as my parents did? I wanted to be loved, but I had a deep anxiety I was missing something or not able to give what was needed, without any idea what precisely it was. How is it possible to trust when you have never been given any reason to trust? All I knew for certain was that the abuse had to be all my fault.

I know I have left a lot of emotional wreckage in my path, some of which I deeply regret. However, I have no regrets over leaving what I can now see were the sort of destructive relationships that I was familiar with. Thinking about it as I write, I still can't work out how Tony and I managed to make our marriage work, given that he also had his own emotional issues. However, from what he told me, he had a relatively happy childhood. He was close to his grandfather, Robert Thompson, and was doted on by his mother, yet he spent most of his adult life shunning responsibility and commitment. At the first whiff of cordite he used to head off, taking the easy option of running away. We both had to learn not to panic and to figure out and accept the sort of levels of unwelcome, thoughtless or ill-tempered behaviour that are pretty much standard in any relationship. Our world was not about to collapse, as nothing is ever perfect – and people who claim never to argue must lead boring lives! So, our relationship worked because we decided it would and because we loved each other. He protected me from my demons and soothed my fears, while I recognised his vulnerabilities.

From the beginning, our marriage was predicated on the basis that this was the last chance for both of us to have a successful and lasting partnership. We promised each other that, no matter what, we would stick together. It goes without saying that over the years this promise was tested to breaking point, but somehow we always managed to work through any crisis, often with gritted teeth and an obstinate refusal to give in. We were both stubborn, even pig-headed at times, but I was definitely more stubborn than him. I can take a lot of hassle before I decide enough is enough and then, no matter what, I will not be budged. It was only as adults my sons realised the word 'sunshine' was not a negative term, as my default, truly hacked-off phrase when they were children was: 'OK, sunshine, are you really trying to make me angry?' I never used 'sunshine' with Tony though he would tease me about it, but he did come up against that same brick wall and then it was another clash of wills.

It was not just living with each other that we had to navigate, it was also becoming stepparents. Tony became a stepfather for the first time to my two youngest boys, Sam and Will. My older sons, Tom and Matthew, were off doing their own thing by then. Tom had decided to train as an officer with the Royal Fleet Auxiliary. He was part of the support fleet for the British Forces during the Iraq War in 2003. Then, he was on the bridge of RFA *Bayleaf*, supplying diesel and jet fuel to NATO and coalition warships. Needless to say, I became an anxious mess, like so many other parents and families whose children were stationed in the Gulf at that time. I made so many deals with God during this period, I am in hock to Him for the next millennium. Later, in the run-up to the 2005 general election, Tony and I were in Blackpool, campaigning. Tony Blair was deeply unpopular at this time because of the government's decision to go to war in Iraq and a man came up to us and spat on me. Besides being completely disgusted, I had to hang on tight to my Tony to prevent him from punching the man, much as he deserved it. He settled for a short shouting match before our colleagues hustled us into a nearby cafe, so I could get cleaned up and we could all have a calming cup of tea. Thank goodness for wet wipes.

My son Matthew has always been one of a kind, never wanting to be tied by the routine and demands of a regular job. He was content to do his own thing, happy to touch base every so often. Tony and I visited him a few times in Paris and once Tony could no longer fly, we opted for the Eurostar instead. In fact, the Eurostar always proved a great adventure and much easier than a plane when it came to getting Tony on and off it.

Naturally, there were challenges to our new roles as stepparents as Tony could become jealous easily of my sons, but for me this was a non-negotiable area. His jealousy was his problem, not mine or my sons', and he was never to try to make me choose between them. That was the only thing that would have been a marriage-breaker. However, having only daughters himself, Tony loved having boys in the house and a rapport formed between them through their shared love of sport. Will was keen on football and played for the junior team in Glossop where we lived. Tony would take him to training at the aptly named Cemetery Road pitch. It is on the top of a hill and in winter it was freezing, and they would come home half perished. He also ferried Will to his matches, standing on the edge of the pitch and chatting with the other parents; he and Will would then dissect the game on their way home in the car. Tony was thrilled when, several years later, Will was spotted by a Blackburn Rovers scout when playing in a university match. All those late-winter afternoons up at Cemetery Road were obviously paying off. He made it all the way to the last round, but didn't make the final selection. Still, it was a brilliant achievement.

For Sam, it was cricket; and he and Tony would go to Old Trafford to watch Lancashire play. One evening, when they arrived home from a match, Tony couldn't wait to tell me the story of how Sam had caught a ball and thrown it back. A little while later a man had appeared, shuffling down the row to Sam. He had been impressed by Sam's return and wanted to know if he would like to train at the club. Of course, Sam said yes, but it was Tony who was overcome with the romance of this *Boys' Own* story. Sam continued to play cricket until he went to university, but then other pursuits became much more interesting.

The fly in the ointment in this sporting heaven was the football teams they supported. As someone who was born and brought up in south Manchester, there was never any question about who I would support – and my commitment to Manchester United was obviously passed through the umbilical cord to my sons. For Tony, brought up in Liverpool where United are anathema, his club was Liverpool. The only time he wasn't concerned about how the team were doing in the league was at the end of his life, when dementia erased his memory. However, before this, the three of them were happy to put aside this rivalry when the occasion demanded.

During the 1998–9 football season, when United won the treble, Tony and I were crossing the concourse at Euston station when we bumped into the then manager of United, Alex Ferguson. We were on our way to a dinner held by the *Tribune* magazine while Fergie was meeting up with his team ahead of the FA Cup Final – we had by then already won the Premier League. It was a very exciting moment for me and one of the few occasions in my life when I have been rendered almost speechless, but Tony was the one who remembered to get Fergie's autograph for Will. Just before the UEFA Champions League final, I was in Prague to complete some research on my doctorate thesis, leaving Tony in charge of an excited Sam and Will and preparations for watching the match. I phoned from Prague, where I had heard the match was going badly for United. All three of the boys, Tony included, were distraught. But, of course, they ended the evening roaring in triumph, more of the male-bonding type stuff.

Will was nine years old when I met Tony, so they spent a long time living together, although I would sometimes have to mediate between them, Will inevitably being closer to his own dad. In the very beginning, Tony's youngest daughter, Jo, also spent quite a lot of time with us. She was a little younger than Will and the novelty of their relationship – my two boys weren't used to sisters and Jo wasn't used to brothers – helped the three of them get on well together. Sadly, it didn't last as Tony's divorce became increasingly bitter and Jo spent less and less time with us. So, despite the difficult moments and the tension that created, it was with Will rather than with Jo that Tony spent more time.

Once, during a fallow period for Tony, he was offered a role in *Owd Bob,* a film that his former partner Julie Allan was helping to produce. He hadn't seen her since the day he came home to find she had gone back to America, taking their children with her. This contact came completely out of the blue and he was dubious about accepting the role, suspicious and nervous of her motives. Eventually, needing the money, he decided to take the work and Will went with him to the Isle of Man, where the film was being shot, to keep Tony company on what might have been enemy territory. Will was only eleven at the time, so being on a film set was an exciting experience for him anyway and something different to do during the long summer holidays.

Sam, five years older than Will, had a close relationship with Tony. Sam liked music and he liked to play it loudly. One track that always stuck in Tony's head because we heard it so many times was the Travis song 'Why Does it

Always Rain on Me?', which soon became Tony's phrase for things not going to plan. When Sam started playing Jimi Hendrix we were both startled. Sam was even more startled that Tony and I had heard of him because, you know, what do parents know about such things? Tony was able to tell him his story about meeting Hendrix and listening to him play when he first arrived in London. Sam was suitably impressed, as was the broadcaster and journalist Andy Kershaw when I boastfully told him the same story not so long ago. I feel it is my duty to repeat some of Tony's best stories occasionally now he no longer can.

Sam asked Tony to give a reading at his wedding. Unfortunately, as can sometimes happen, things went wrong after that, especially once Sam's first child, Harry, was born. For reasons unknown to us Tony and I were gradually cut out of their lives and unable to see their children – Isolde was born a few years later. I know this is something that happens to grandparents, but there is no comfort in the crowd, and we were hurt and at a loss as to what had caused this behaviour. Things became much more difficult for Tony as his dementia worsened and he would frequently ask why he didn't see Sam. I don't know how often I had to explain Sam was busy with his own family. But, of course, each time I told him, it was like the first time as he couldn't remember being told before – which meant he was repeatedly upset by the news. Personally, I believe no matter the issues, Tony had dementia and Sam should have made more time for him. He did visit Tony about a week before he died, but as with some of his daughters, Tony didn't remember who he was.

It's strange yet true that even after twenty-something years of living with their father, I don't really know his daughters. What I do know is that despite a long history of abandoned women and daughters and everything he may have said to the contrary, Tony did want his children to love him; his only caveat being that it had to be on his terms, although it was never clear what exactly those terms were. I tried over the years to build bridges between them, but eventually realised that his children wanted him, not me, to do that. Tony didn't help his own cause either by not making any real effort. He believed that his children should come to him as their father, not the other way round. He could be a complete blockhead at times.

Of course, I accompanied Tony when he was invited to the big occasions in his daughters' lives. I was with him at the Royal Festival Hall in London, for instance, the night Labour won a landslide victory in the 1997 election. Nothing could ever quite reach the dizzying excitement of that event, but there were family weddings to enjoy.

Tony's daughter Lauren married the actor Craig Darby in 2001. Initially, Lauren had not invited her father, as they were not speaking at the time. But *Hello* magazine, who were paying for the event, wanted him there to be included in the photo shoot. It was all a little awkward and I blotted my copybook further by taking a call from my son Tom during the speeches. He was away at sea at the time and I was getting a little anxious as I had not heard from him in a while, so I didn't want to miss the opportunity to speak to him. During our conversation, I looked up to see all the other wedding guests staring at me. Lauren was giving her speech and had mentioned me. Glancing across, she'd spotted me on the phone and not unreasonably made a crack about it. It was embarrassing, but we were seated well away from the top table, so I don't think too many people would have been disturbed by my whispered conversation. I suppose I could have left the room, but then that might have been seen as even more offensive.

When Emma, Lauren's sister, married Tony Roch (yet another Tony) on Hydra, one of the Greek islands, it was a glorious event. It is such a pretty island, a perfect place for the wedding, which took place on a beach. My Tony performed the traditional dad part of giving the bride away. I think this was the one and only time he played that role and he was thrilled. From then on, it was his grandchildren's weddings that we attended, and he wasn't short of a grandchild or two – with ten grandchildren in total.

Euan Blair, Tony's eldest grandson, got married in September 2013. This time the wedding took place in the slightly less exotic location of the Blairs' family home in Buckinghamshire. My Tony was, at Cherie's insistence, kitted out with a new suit, but along the way someone had made the rash decision of allowing him to choose his own tie. It was awful, but he was happy and it was only later when he saw the photographs he demanded to know why I had let him wear it. The wedding was, of course, a huge family affair, but even then Tony was struggling to remember who people were. This didn't stop him enjoying himself, though.

The wedding of Tony's second grandson, Nicky, took place in July 2015 with the ceremony again being held at South Pavilion. It was another beautiful wedding, but Tony's memory and health were considerably worse by this point. He found the whole day something of a struggle. I was really quite concerned about him and we left the celebrations early, as did Gale, Cherie and Lyndsey's mum. If anything, I think Gale was more tired and confused than Tony. She was by this time living in a care home, where she died in June the following year.

Given the distant relationship I had with Tony's children, it came as a great relief that some of them were really supportive when he died. Cherie and Lyndsey gave me the most help in the weeks leading up to Tony's funeral despite the fact that my last real contact with Lyndsey had been a few years earlier, when we had had a furious row conducted by email. The row might perhaps have had an enduring influence on some of our exchanges, but happily it didn't and afterwards, whenever she phoned to speak to her dad, we would make polite enquiries about each other before I passed the phone over to her father. After he died, she contacted me every day and when necessary in the round-robin emails between her sisters, she pointed out that it was my role to organise the funeral. I was the one who knew what their father's wishes were. Her help was timely. At his funeral, tucked under her bright red coat, Lyndsey wore a Liverpool football club scarf. A discreet but touching way to honour her dad.

I think a lot of the difficulties between Tony's daughters and me arose from what I felt was a lack of understanding and support. Cherie would always help if I asked, but I didn't like to ask (sometimes feeling as if I hadn't explored other alternatives sufficiently). I didn't want her to think I was using her as the easy option. This was far from the case, as I would do anything to avoid having to ask and squirmed inwardly any time I had to write a 'please help' email.

In the earlier days when her dad was ill enough to need help and support but not bad enough for respite in a care home, Cherie would have him to stay at her South Pavilion home near Oxford. This would give me a few days off to have a break. South Pavilion is lovely and spacious and has the benefit of big gardens, which meant Tony was unlikely to wander far. He liked the countryside, and this was a great substitute. One of the other great advantages was in the form of Ann and Andy, who ran the house. Tony and Andy were good friends and Ann made sure he was well fed. Cherie offered me practical support, which I appreciated. But then, as there was so little contact with the rest of his daughters during his illness, how could they have known about our situation or what was needed?

When Tony Blair stood in the 1992 General Election for the parliamentary seat of Sedgefield, my Tony and his then wife Pat Phoenix campaigned for him. When Tony Blair won the seat, he and Cherie bought a house in the constituency. Tony told me Pat was delighted to give them some of her own things to help furnish the house, as this gave her the golden opportunity to go out and buy new furniture for their home. Being such a political animal, my Tony was thrilled when Tony Blair got into Parliament and continued to support him through every general election he fought. Tony was, of course, fit to burst with pride when the Blairs moved into 10 Downing Street after the landslide victory of '97. Tony and I became fairly frequent visitors to Number 10, but it was family events at Chequers that were the great highlights.

One of them was Cherie's fiftieth birthday party, memorable for the demonstration at the gates of the house by the pro-hunting lobby, who were upset by the government's proposal to ban fox hunting. While we waited in the queue of cars for a decision to be made about how to get guests into the house – security, quite reasonably in the circumstances, not wanting to open the gates – Tony decided he needed to pee. He got out of the car and went to speak to a policeman, who pointed him in the direction of some bushes and who then decided that he too needed to pee and went with Tony. I watched in horrified fascination, knowing full well that the *Daily Mail* would have far more fun with a headline about Tony Booth disappearing into bushes with a policeman than they would with any crummy old piece about fox hunters.

Eventually we were all dispersed to various points within a short radius of Chequers to wait for an escort to take us to the house along a circuitous back route. Cherie was determined her milestone birthday party was going ahead – and quite right too, it was a great do. As she was then a big fan of *Strictly Come Dancing*, Cherie was hoping to persuade the cricketer Mark Ramprakash, a recent contestant, to come and take part in some ballroom dancing. He wasn't available so she had settled for Anton du Beke who, unsurprisingly, was not terribly happy with the number of times his toes were trodden on by various eager women.

For me and Tony, one of the best moments to come out of his son-in-law being Prime Minister happened in 2002. As part of the celebrations to mark the Commonwealth Games in Manchester that year, Cherie was asked to help launch the Literature of the Commonwealth Festival at a gala dinner. She invited her dad and me along to the event.

At the meal, I was seated one person away from the South African High Commissioner, Lindiwe Mabuza. She looked beautiful in full African dress, but it was her ebony necklace that was particularly magnificent. At some point in the evening we began chatting – I think I commented on her necklace – and our conversation went on from there as we exchanged stories about our children. As she had been an ANC representative during the unspeakable apartheid regime, she was an interesting person to listen to, particularly her story about being based in New York and asked by CNN to comment on Nelson Mandela's release from prison. She explained she had not been expecting to be so overcome as she watched the television footage of him walking out of jail.

As the dinner ended and people started to circulate, we began talking again and I told her how much I would like to meet Nelson Mandela. Asking if Tony would like to meet him too, she promised to arrange something for the next time Mr Mandela was in Britain. I thought it was a kind offer, but given how busy he would be, I didn't really think it would be possible. However, a few weeks later, there was a telephone call from the High Commission to make arrangements for Tony and me to have morning coffee with Nelson Mandela. It was an amazing and emotional experience and another time in my life when I was completely stuck for words, although fortunately Tony was, as usual, completely at ease. I did eventually manage to join in the chat. The photograph of the three of us still hangs on the sitting-room wall.

The connection with South Africa continued when in 2006 Tony appeared in a short film, *Blinding Lights* produced by Rosemary Boateng. At the time, Sam was home after a brief, unhappy period at the University of Leicester. After a suitable period of loafing around as he recovered his equilibrium, I decided it was time he made new plans. He wasn't yet keen to go back into education, so I suggested maybe volunteering in the developing world could be a good strategy: it would help to confirm his moral views whilst also giving him first-hand experience about the economics and politics of those countries. Now, Rosemary is the sister of Paul Boateng, who at the time was the UK's High Commissioner to South Africa. Tony had got on well with Rosemary and thanks to their help, Sam became a volunteer worker in a township in the Eastern Cape. Tony was convinced it would be the making of him, whilst I was not entirely sure he would cope with the challenge. I thought he would be on a flight home within a few days, but I'm pleased to say Tony was right.

It is natural as parents to want better for our children than we had ourselves. I sometimes wonder if we have not gone too far with this aspiration, giving them nothing much to work for or to aim for. Have we made it too easy for them?

I know Sam was shocked at the realities of life in a South African township. Young children were regularly sleeping rough, but there was a local woman who took some of them in. She had no means of support, relying entirely on donations. Sam and a colleague decided to take food to her and the children. They bought a good supply of the usual heavy-duty dry goods such as pasta and rice, as well as fruit and vegetables. They also bought sweets, assuming they would be as much a treat for the children as they had been for him and his friend when they were little. Sam phoned me later to tell me the children had ignored the sweets, instead making a rush for the fruit, as that was their special treat. My son came home with a heightened awareness of what he had and the opportunities life had given him. On his return, he applied to Manchester Metropolitan University to study English. His experience in South Africa had given him focus and purpose.

Sam was not the only one thinking about his future: it was something Tony and I were also discussing, particularly after we holidayed to Ireland more and more. It was a country that, given our shared Irish heritage, we both had something of a yearning for.

The first time we went to Ireland we arrived in Dublin during the rush hour, but Tony insisted there was no need to worry as he knew his way around. Things were fine until we reached St Stephen's Green, which was when I realised Tony didn't know the city as well as he claimed. As the one driving the car, I became increasingly frustrated and Tony was getting bad tempered – a potentially combustible situation. Eventually, via an extended trip through a council estate and a brief, unhelpful period of not talking to each other, we did find our hotel on Lansdowne Road.

This initial hiccup did not put us off and we visited Ireland several times, exploring as far west as Kerry. We stayed in Kildare with Tony's friends William and Susan. William is the legendary G.W. Robinson who famously rode Mill House to victory in the 1963 Cheltenham Gold Cup. Tony loved horse racing, being initiated as a young boy into the horse-betting habit by his grandfather, Robert Thompson. When I first met Tony fifty years later, he still had an account with the betting shop William Hill. Being able to talk horses and horse racing with William was Tony's idea of bliss, as unlike his late wife, Pat Phoenix, with whom Tony owned horses, I know nothing about the sport and was therefore not really worth talking to. I far preferred Susan's garden and chickens to looking at horses. They are a bit in the big side for me and I'm scared of them biting.

We made the move to Ireland in 2003, looking for a slower pace of life. The election of the Labour government in 1997 had impacted on our lives in ways I could not have expected. Things could get a little crazy at times, such as when Leo, Cherie's youngest son, was born in May 2000. I opened our back door to find the press waiting to speak to Tony about the event. Of course, he took it all in his stride. I was less pleased, particularly when in order to get my children to school that morning, we had to cut through several of our neighbours' gardens to avoid photographers. Eventually even Tony, who loved being the centre of attention, could see the attraction of a quieter life.

At the same time as looking for a home, we looked at schools for Will for his sixth-form education. After investigating possible options, Will and I decided it would be better for him to stay in England with his father. This meant that for the first time Tony and I would be living alone together; something that in retrospect turned out to be really important, given what we were later to endure. We moved knowing it would not be for ever, as we would at some point run out of money, but it is true it's always the things you don't do that you regret the most. We took the plunge and it was one of the best decisions we ever made.

3.

First signs

The first signs of Tony's dementia passed me by, probably because I wasn't looking for symptoms. I was more concerned about the effect his smoking was having on his heart and lungs. It was cancer that was my main health concern for him. He was certainly becoming more forgetful and confused, but I put that down to his increasing age. The idea he might have dementia never crossed my mind, so I wasn't looking for possible indicators or warning signs. I think few of us these days would recognise the onset of dementia.

Thinking back, the only previous experience I had of someone with dementia was my great-grandmother, Lizzie Buckley. I was only seven when she died, so my recollection is limited to an old lady who lived in the house of my maternal grandmother, Kathleen. I was far too young to realise the implications of the situation and, with the indifference of youth, the difficulties my grandmother faced. At that time, the assumption and reality was that Lizzie would be cared for at home even if she was, as my grandmother said, 'gaga'.

Lizzie wore mostly black, spent her days in a chair by the fire and, when she was not asleep, would terrorise anyone near her. Her fox fur hung in the hallway and she would threaten her great-grandchildren with being bitten by it if we annoyed her. We had to be very quiet – we were almost too scared to breathe. We were, though, expected to treat her with the same consideration and respect we'd been taught to give any adult. Her frailty was no excuse to sideline her from a central role in her family. Eventually, Lizzie's bed was moved downstairs into the parlour – my gran's best room where troublesome and inquisitive children were not allowed. She eventually died in her bed, a tiny, shrunken woman.

Tony never threatened me with a fox fur. Instead, as I've mentioned, he would threaten me with his 'lawyers', Cherie and Lyndsey. I would shrug my shoulders, confident in the knowledge that it would get him precisely nowhere.

I am fortunate to have known and been loved by Kathleen Buckley. My grandmother's influence on my outlook on life has been invaluable and lifelong. Widowed during the Second World War, she was left with three small children to bring up. That was when Lizzie moved in to share the house and help look after the children. My gran worked in a munitions factory in Trafford Park during the war. Afterwards, she held down three cleaning jobs – too proud to rely on handouts from anyone, including the state. So much so, she didn't even claim her widow's pension. Years later, when my uncle discovered this and made a retrospective claim, she had enough in back payments to buy the terraced house she had been renting for decades. Like so many women of her time and generation, Kathleen Buckley was a heroine. Tough, determined and big-hearted, she drilled into me the importance of not wasting time and energy moaning and crying in the face of problems and difficulties. Her attitude was to get on with it and sort it out. I can still hear her voice when I sometimes struggle to face up to major events such as moving house, or, more profoundly, when I was coping with Tony's diagnosis, needing all my love and strength for the years ahead.

Moving house is a big step. Moving house and country is a major step. It goes almost without saying that our move to Ireland entailed various traumas and high dramas for Tony and me to navigate, along with the more usual negotiations and compromises a decision like this involves.

Things started reasonably enough as we made arrangements for the ferry to Dublin and I began looking online at potential properties. It had to be me as Tony was a committed Luddite all his life and never got the hang of mobile phones, let alone computers. There were two possible reasons for this. Firstly, he was something of a lazy fellow and one of his key philosophies was never to stand when you can sit and never to sit when you can lie down. So, given that I'm computer literate, really why would he need to bother? Secondly, as I search my memory for clues, was his technophobia hiding yet another missed dementia indicator, the fading ability to learn new skills?

Our price range and preferences in terms of what we wanted – mountains, lakes, close to the coast – made the north-west of Ireland the obvious choice. We drove up from Dublin to Carrick-on-Shannon. I had read in one of the guidebooks that there was a good bed-and-breakfast in the town, Hollywell. We tended to stay in B&Bs rather than hotels as usually the quality of the breakfast was considerably better and privacy easier to come by. A full cooked breakfast was a treat we always enjoyed. We also thought Carrick-on-Shannon would make a good base for exploring the area. However, we hadn't made a reservation at Hollywell bed-and-breakfast, something I wouldn't be so laissez-faire about in the future. Organisation was crucial when taking Tony anywhere for my sanity and his wellbeing. Fortunately, the owners Tom and Rosie Maher had rooms available. We were shown upstairs and left to settle in.

As we pottered around, hanging up clothes and making a pot of tea, we could hear what we thought might be a slightly animated discussion going on downstairs. The sound was muffled, so we couldn't work out what exactly was going on. The next thing was a knock on our bedroom door. Tom was standing there. He wanted us to move across the landing into a larger room at the front of the house where he thought we would be more comfortable. Tony told him we were fine, but Tom was keen for us to move. Rather than cause any fuss – we did not know what had been decided downstairs – with Tom's help, we carried our things into the other bedroom.

He then invited us to the sitting-room for tea. It turned out the discussion we'd heard was about whether Tony was Tony Booth the actor. If indeed he was *the* Tony Booth then maybe he should have a bigger room. To be on the safe side, even though they thought Tony Booth was unlikely to be in Carrick-on-Shannon, Rosie and Tom decided to move us across the landing. We had a lovely time chatting to them over several pots of tea. Rosie and Tom became good friends to us and helped us enormously with support and advice during our move to Ireland and throughout our time there.

Searching for a new home is stressful even when you have some idea of what you want. Finding that ideal place is the problem. Initially, Tony and I headed south from Carrick-on-Shannon with great optimism. Optimism that was soon dashed. Like most potential house buyers, we became somewhat cynical about estate agent blurbs. Irish estate agents appear to have the same imaginative capacities as their British counterparts. The writers are clearly under the influence of something. 'Needs some work' means the roof has fallen in. 'Has a few damp problems' reveals the carpet squelches as you walk across it. 'Needs renovating' – and you'll find the roof has fallen in, nature has taken back control and the building has no connections to any mains services. Cracking that code was a vital first step.

One house we looked at was incredibly damp. A carpet squelcher. The thing that reduced me to helpless laughter, though, was the plaster statue of the Virgin and baby Jesus. It was about eighteen inches tall and stood on the mantelpiece in the middle room. I have never seen such a battered Virgin. Lumps were missing. As I recall, baby Jesus had lost his nose. I was laughing so hard I thought I might wet myself. Hysteria had clearly set in. Tony, by now cross and fed up after several viewings, had refused to come further than the front door. We made our excuses and left, explaining we were too tired to continue our exploration. Sometimes, things don't always go as you hope or plan.

Nothing caught our eye. Were we being too picky? I realised Tony was increasingly stressed and tired, and rather than expand our search as the television experts advise, we chose to focus and look only at places we thought might be 'definite maybes'. Breezing along, I missed potential symptoms of dementia. I thought Tony was simply getting bored, which was highly probable, but I did not particularly pick up on his lack of focus and his confusion and the fact that I was expecting him to absorb too much information. I didn't realise how tiring my bombardment of enthusiasm was for him. I would have a lot to learn.

Food was eventually to become an enormous issue in our lives, but back then it was a way of breaking up the day – trying not to irritate or exhaust Tony too much. Little and often was the answer, as we stopped to discuss the houses we had seen and what to do next. To be honest, I found this frustrating – I just wanted to crack on and find somewhere – but when our fun and excitement gauge dipped to zero, lunch was called for. As Tony's Alzheimer's progressed and he was eating less and less, no matter what I said or did, meal times became a flashpoint for tension. Not even little and often worked.

On the third day of our trip we found the house we wanted to live in, in Moneygashel. It was the first one we saw that day. We went on to view a few more, but then came back to it. It was a genuine discovery, standing in an acre of grounds, with a small wood across the lane that ran in front of the house and magnificent views across to Cuilcagh Mountain. We weren't fazed that it would need work. My greatest concern was it was painted pink. Not just any pink, but cerise. I don't like pink and cerise was beyond the pale. I tried to explain to Tony and Sean, the estate agent, that I couldn't possibly live in a cerise house, but my concerns were lost on them. They both just stared slack-jawed at me. 'Well, it could be painted,' Sean suggested diplomatically. Tony just said I was bonkers. Tony and I bought the house. Despite the cerise it had potential and no squelchy floors.

We then went home to Broadbottom to sell our old house, which was bought very quickly by a young couple in the neighbourhood. The principle thing that sold the house for us was the garden: being the keen gardener that I am, I had put much love and devotion into it. Leaving the house was a big wrench as we were also moving away from our lovely neighbours. Harold at number 10 had helped Will to make a bird table for the garden. I think it was the only thing from the garden I took to Ireland, as handmade gifts from our children are precious. I have an old laundry box upstairs full of cards and other bits and pieces made by my sons when they were at primary school. Goodness knows what they make of it all. Yet another of their mother's many eccentricities!

That summer held other things in store for me, including the somewhat shocking revelation that Tony had another daughter. I was aware of his other seven children, but Lucy had been living in Australia for many years. Her mother, Annabelle, had moved to Australia when Lucy was very young and Lucy was now married with a young son of her own, Peter. Through an intermediary, Annabelle and Lucy contacted Tony and Cherie. They wanted to connect with the family they had never met. I had no idea how to react when Tony first showed me the letter. To be honest, my first thought was what else had he not told me – especially after he confessed he had always known of Lucy's existence. Not acknowledging or even telling me about a further child was something of a major omission. If that was what it was.

It was arranged that the three Australians would go first to Downing Street to meet Cherie and then travel north to Broadbottom to stay with us. I was far from convinced this was a good idea, but Tony was determined it would happen. Obviously, there was a level of guilty conscience on his part for his past neglect of Lucy, but I felt anxious about having complete strangers in our home. There was an initial compromise whereby they stayed with friends of ours for a few days until we got to know them a little better, before coming to stay with us.

As Tony always loved being the centre of attention, when Annabelle and Lucy suggested he accompany them to meet their friends and family, he was off like a shot. Why stick with the humdrum and everyday at home when he could go off and be feted? To this day, I have no idea where he went. I was so angry I changed the locks. He further compounded his sins by not telephoning me once during the several days he was away. What was the old fool doing? We were supposed to be moving to Ireland and there he was, at seventy years old, swanning around the country with a former girlfriend.

On his return, I stood and watched as he attempted to unlock the half-glazed back door. It took a while for him to realise his key wouldn't work. Increasingly belligerent, he demanded to be let in.

'Not until you stop shouting. Then I'll open the door,' I said.

Of course, he did not want to give in. But neither would I. Tony was quick to fly into hot-tempered, theatrical rages, but – as I've mentioned – I can be very stubborn. He didn't have a chance.

Eventually he said, 'Steph, please let me in.'

When I opened the door, he walked in, yelling. This was his default defence position: refusing to acknowledge any mistakes he'd made or apologise. He argued that it was my fault and that he would be moving to Ireland with or without me.

'Fine,' I said, walking away.

Nobody in the house, Will, Sam or I, would talk to him. I also refused to cook for him and he was left to sort himself out. This was torture and he survived for, at most, thirty-six hours. It was that long because he took to his bed for eighteen of them. He struggled on a little while more before caving in and telling me how much he loved me, what a mistake he had made and how the only thing he wanted to do was to move to our little house in Ireland together. My stubbornness has, in the past, led me into all sorts of trouble and situations I have regretted. This time, it was useful in demonstrating to Tony that he had gone too far and I would not tolerate his embarrassing and thoughtless behaviour. I have never once considered putting this incident down to encroaching dementia.

Eventually, Tony and I boarded the ferry from Holyhead on our journey to our new home in Ireland, each in our own car, the two cats and two dogs travelling with me. When we arrived in Dublin it was dark and we'd hit the rush hour. Although planning to travel in convoy, we were soon separated and I began to worry if Tony would find his way to Moneygashel. As he didn't use sat nav, he would have to rely on map reading. This did not fill me with hope.

I arrived at the house first. There was no sign of Tony, so I unloaded the animals and fed them. We had planned our first night at a bed-and-breakfast in Blacklion, a small town not far away. Leaving the animals in the house, I drove to Blacklion to see if Tony was there. He wasn't. It was now more than an hour since I had arrived. I went across to the Garda office to see if there were any reports of a man in a car with British plates, driving around lost. Again, nothing, but the Garda said he would radio his colleagues to keep an eye out for him. I went back to Moneygashel and waited. It was late at night and the house was freezing. By now really worried, I returned to Blacklion to find Tony at the bed-and-breakfast, enjoying a cup of tea. He had got lost and been brought in by a Garda. In the end it didn't matter, we were finally there.

One of the issues we had discussed before moving was Tony's dope habit. On moving to Ireland, I was clear he would have to stop smoking. As we would be living in an isolated area close to the border with the North, my major concern was that I didn't want questionable types offering drugs on our doorstep. Who knew where that might lead? Peace and harmony were on offer – and Tony agreed. As far as I am aware, Tony kept his promise. I believe he didn't smoke dope after we moved, but what he got up to when he was working in England was anybody's guess.

The questionable men turned up anyway. Not offering drugs, but on a manhunt. A few weeks after we moved in, Tony and I were standing in our driveway, chatting to a neighbour, when a large black car with blacked-out windows pulled up. Three men stepped out of the car. They were big blokes in black suits, crisp, white shirts and ties and dark glasses. They were immaculate. It was like something out of *Reservoir Dogs*. Who on earth were they and what were they doing here? They stood by their car with no intention, it seemed, of approaching us. We all looked at each other in surprise and eventually I walked over to them.

'Can I help you?'

One of the men mentioned a name and asked me if I knew this person.

'No.'

'You must know him. You live round here.'

'No. We've only just moved in and don't know anybody, really,' I helpfully responded.

They stood and stared at us for a few more moments, then got back in their car and drove away.

As I walked back to the house, our neighbour said to me, 'You are one crazy woman. They're Belfast mafia. I can't believe they've just driven away.'

I don't know how true that was, but even the mafia should display some good manners. The man in black had failed to take his sunglasses off to speak to me.

It turned out they were looking for someone who had gone to make his fortune as a hairdresser in Belfast. Unfortunately for him, he'd borrowed money from the wrong people. I do not know what happened to this individual and the men never came back. Thankfully. I may not have been quite so brave, or foolhardy, another time.

As we settled in, we busied ourselves unpacking and organising, all those time-consuming and intermittently pleasurable activities of setting up home. At the same time, Tony continued to commute back and forth to the UK for work, which was still fairly steady. He was working on television programmes including *Mersey Beat*, *EastEnders*, *Doctors* and *Dalziel and Pascoe*. Television acting meant there would be retakes when necessary, which was helpful, and as Tony no longer had big parts, it was relatively easy for him to learn his lines. Even as I write this I am astounded I failed to recognise there might have been anything more serious than 'senior moments'. Having said that, I do not know what I could have done. Tony was happy. Any intervention from me would have made him angry and uncertain.

Living in Ireland was the happiest time of our life together. The strain of the baggage we had each brought to our marriage began to slip away. We now had time to remember and enjoy what had first brought us together. Tony and I were so lucky to have found each other at this relatively late point in our lives.

When he was away, I would stay in Ireland with the dogs and cats, happily pottering around and going for walks. There was always plenty of light, even in deep mid-winter. Without light pollution, the night skies were extraordinary and awe-inspiring. I had no idea there were so many stars and how easy it could be to spot the various constellations. Going outside, lying flat on the ground and staring up at the sky was one of the most amazing experiences of my life. It almost felt as if I were being drawn up into the heavens. The world seemed a beautiful place.

We had clearly made the right decision, but I still needed to find work. My *Irish Times* column was the result of my meeting Dr Pat Harrold when I registered with the local GP surgery in Blacklion. I mentioned an idea I had about writing a newspaper column that described what it was like for an urban English couple moving to rural Ireland. It turned out Pat knew the Features Editor at the *Irish Times*, Deirdre Falvey, and he offered to telephone her to discuss my idea with her. That same afternoon, I had a call from the *Irish Times*, which was when my association with the newspaper started. I had no particular remit, I could write what I wanted – and so I did.

It was lovely to receive messages from people who were touched by the column. I had a lot of emails from America – particularly from people who had family and friends local to me. One woman from New York told me it was the first thing she read on the bus to work, to find out what was going on at home. We once had a visitor from America turn up on our doorstep. After the initial confusion of why he was there, we invited him in for tea, cake and a chat.

Tony was always very proud of the fact I wrote for the *Irish Times*. It is a prestigious paper and he never failed to inform people of this fact. It was through writing for the newspaper that I met the Sinn Féin politicians Martin McGuinness and Gerry Adams. We had been invited to the University of Derry for the Tip O'Neill peace lecture, given that year by Hillary Clinton. Before the lecture started, people were milling about, chatting and drinking tea and coffee. As usual, when everyone started to move into the lecture theatre, Tony needed a last-minute wee. Standing waiting for him, I noticed someone approaching me out of the corner of my eye. It was Martin McGuinness. He wanted to shake my hand and tell me how much he enjoyed reading my column, but more importantly how he thought my and Tony's move to Ireland had contributed to normalising the situation there. I hope he was not simply being polite and that in some very small way we did help with the peace process. Martin then took me by the elbow and said, 'Come and meet Gerry.'

I was standing talking to them when Tony eventually reappeared after what must have been the longest wee on record. His face was an absolute picture when he saw who I was chatting to. Of course, I introduced him and we all then moved on to take our seats for the lecture. 'Jesus wept, woman. I leave you alone for five minutes and come back to find you talking to the IRA,' was all Tony had time to say before the lecture started. I suppose it was an indication of how far the peace process had travelled that it seemed, and was, an entirely reasonable thing to do.

We were invited to take part in the Cavan Literary Festival. Elaine Lennon, who was then the arts organiser for Cavan, contacted Tony some months prior to the event to ask if he would give a reading from his autobiography. He agreed, barring acting commitments, to take part. When Tony told me about this conversation, he neglected to mention that Elaine had also asked if I would be willing to facilitate a panel discussion during the festival. Yet he had readily agreed on my behalf. When she telephoned me some while later, I was a little unclear as to what the conversation was about. Once the confusion was cleared (Elaine not unreasonably assumed my husband might have mentioned her request to me), I was delighted to be involved. My contribution was on the opening night, chairing a panel that included the

Irish Times columnist and writer John Waters, the columnist and social diarist John McEntee and the novelist Evelyn Conlon, editor of *Later On: The Monaghan Bombing Memorial Anthology*. The issue under discussion was politics and storytelling. How far do fact and fiction merge and how can we then know what is true? It was an early debate around the issue of fake news, more chastely referred to in those days as 'storytelling'.

You know those awful, embarrassing moments that can still make you squirm years later? I had one of those moments that evening, involving John Waters. His column used to appear on the page before mine in the *Irish Times*, so if he was on page 9 I would be on 11. As I was introduced to him I said, 'It's lovely to meet you properly, given that I'm underneath you on a Monday.' There was a stunned silence as I began to go crimson with the realisation of what I had just said. Then everybody burst out laughing – apart from John Waters. He was stony-faced. He obviously thought I was an idiot, not worth responding to. I sincerely wished the ground would swallow me up. Fortunately, the panel discussion went well and I managed to hold on to the tattered remains of my dignity.

Tony's book reading went well the next evening. It was a packed session and nobody seemed to notice the occasions when he went off-piste, telling stories rather than reading from his book. Whilst I noticed as I had helped him pick out the pages to read from, I did not make anything of it. It was simply Tony being Tony, having a good time and abandoning the agreed format. He was an excellent raconteur.

What I had begun to notice was that Tony, never a good driver, was becoming less skilful. Nothing too serious, but it was a little concerning at times. There was the time when Sam had been over to visit for a few days and he needed a lift back to Dublin airport. Tony insisted he would drive him – I think he wanted to spend a little more time with him. Within half an hour of setting off, they were back. Tony had taken a corner too fast, skidded on some mud, hit a bank and flipped the car over. I was not worried about the car, but I did go screaming mad at Tony for risking my son's life. They were both shaken up, but neither of them was hurt. By a stroke of good fortune, another car had been coming the other way; the couple in the car had stopped to help and dropped them off at the house. Tony's car was retrieved, unbelievably with very little damage to it. But I now began to have little doubts and niggles of worry about Tony's concentration. I began to piece together all the other little moments of forgetfulness and confusion I had not really considered significant. Yet I still did not consider these to be signs of anything more sinister than ageing. My solution was to do most of the driving myself. It took someone more objective to join up the dots for me.

When our friends Jean and John came to stay, it was suggested to me that Tony's symptoms might be caused by something other than his growing older. We have been friends for many years and they could immediately see some things had changed. As a GP, John knew far better than I did what signs to look for. He was of the opinion it might be wise to have Tony checked out, but there was no need to panic.

Jean and John are excellent company. On this occasion, we spent our time together walking in the mountains, then coming home to enjoy cooking food and drinking wine. They loved our house as much as Tony and I did. On one particular evening, while we were chatting and drinking wine, there was a knock on the front door. We all looked at each other. It was a dark winter's night and we did not yet know many local people. When I opened the door, a priest was standing there. His name was Father Michael and he was calling to introduce himself. I ushered him into the kitchen where the peat fire was still burning. I put the kettle on and, excusing myself, went back into the sitting-room where John, Jean and Tony were sat silently. Not wanting to give the priest the wrong impression on first acquaintance, I instructed everyone to hide the wine bottles and glasses.

When I brought Father Michael into the sitting-room with his mug of tea you would have sworn we were joining a teetotallers' group. Settling himself into an armchair, Father Michael seemed oblivious to the slightly awkward atmosphere and began chatting away. Oscar, our black cat, decided to join him, taking the space on the back of his chair. Jean and I were sitting on the couch and after a short while she nudged me in the ribs, rolling her eyes towards the armchair. To my complete mortification, Oscar had fallen deeply in lust. Purring and drooling, she was nuzzling the back of the head of the seemingly oblivious priest. Jean and I shared an agonised look before I took control of the situation and grabbed the cat, lobbing her on to the floor. Stalking away with that huffy, haughty look cats do so well, she went behind the couch. Without batting an eyelid at this intervention, the priest simply carried on chatting.

I had no idea where the glasses and bottles were hidden at this point. But I soon found out when Oscar, in vengeful mode, began pushing them over. As I began thinking vengeful thoughts of my own, to my horror an empty wine bottle rolled out from under the couch. But Father Michael was delighted, saying, 'Oh, that's good. I didn't know you had the hard stuff. I'll take a drop of whiskey, myself.' Things then became very convivial and it was quite late by the time he left.

*

I had taken on board what John had said about Tony, but was happy at first to go with the 'no need to panic' part of his advice. Actors can be odd, egotistical creatures and I can say with some authority that they often appear to inhabit a parallel universe. Inevitable perhaps, given they spend their professional lives pretending to be someone else. This behaviour can spill into their private lives and by this point I was finding it difficult to discern the 'merely eccentric' from behaviour I should be anxious about. Tony was a voracious reader, but I began to realise he was sometimes having trouble differentiating between fact and fiction. He would start a conversation with me which I would be unable to follow, until it became obvious the people he was referring to were characters in a book he was reading. Tony was never one to let the truth get in the way of a good story, but this was different. This was concerning.

That was when I decided to act on John's advice. Tony would have to see a doctor. I had to know what was happening. But getting him to the doctor would be no easy task. He would not go if I told him I was concerned he might have dementia. Dr Pat Harrold had, by then, moved to Tipperary and I didn't know the new doctor very well. I went to see him to talk about Tony and to explain I had devised a cunning plan, which needed his co-operation, to bring Tony to the surgery.

What I wanted to do was to get Tony to the surgery for a physical check-up on the pretext that this was a policy introduced by the Irish government. This was true to a point and knowing Tony was something of a hypochondriac, I was fairly certain he would buy into it. At this point, the doctor was still on board. It was the next part of the plan he baulked at. I convinced myself it was not exactly a lie, but it was certainly being economical with the truth. I wanted the doctor to tell Tony that, as part of this post-age-seventy check-up, the government also had a policy of checking for any deterioration in mental capacity. Carefully not mentioning 'dementia'. The doctor took a great deal of convincing. I had to agree to carry the can for anything that might go wrong before he eventually and reluctantly agreed to my plan.

The checks revealed that physically Tony, apart from a bit of a smoker's cough, was as fit as a fiddle, but the doctor was worried about dementia too, so he referred us to a psychologist in Sligo. Still believing my tale about the government health policy, Tony was happy to go along. There were times when, out of embarrassment, I wished I had not pursued this line of action. Tony's default position, when he was uncertain, was to joke about and tell stories. This made it difficult for the psychologist, who ran various tests over several sessions, to come to any firm conclusions. Tony would not focus on the task in hand. Of course he wouldn't, as the very idea that the tests might reveal a loss of short-term memory was unbearable to him. How would he be able to work if that was the case? He was an actor –

it was who he was – and he never wanted to do or be anything else.

I had also made the psychologist aware of Tony's dope habit. Even though Tony insisted it was irrelevant, when he spoke to me the psychologist was clear it made any diagnosis much more difficult and he could not provide a definitive result. What damage had the drug done to Tony's brain? How many of his current problems were the result of dementia and to what extent was dope responsible for brain-cell destruction? Were the two interlinked? Who knows? I still hung on to the hope that Tony's apparent mental decline was simply the decrepitude of old age.

We went home comforted by the psychologist's indecision and carried on as we were, Tony because he would not – and did not – ever accept he had dementia. He believed that by shutting out the news and employing the sheer force of his will, he would delay, even prevent, the inevitable. For me, it was a strategy of not facing up to the reality of what dementia might bring and whether I could cope with it. We humans – well, me certainly – have an incredible capacity to hope against hope that everything will work out all right in the end. I cannot work out now if I was blasé or simply naive. Perhaps it is a good thing I had no idea what was coming down the track towards us.

4.
Diagnosis

After the first tentative diagnosis, there was no significant development in the symptoms that had initially concerned me. Yes, Tony would get confused and sometimes I had to explain things several times before he understood, but nothing that had too much of an impact on our lives. I made a few adjustments to cope with his behaviour, but everything seemed fine. Given the circumstances, it was easy to convince myself we'd had something of a false alarm.

When, in 2002, he was offered the part of Bottom in *A Midsummer Night's Dream*, my only concern was a stage run that included afternoon matinees several times a week, as well as evening performances, would be too physically demanding. Tony, though, was adamant he wanted to do it and would get angry with me when I questioned the wisdom of his decision. I understood where he was coming from. Theatre had always been his first love.

Tony started his acting career on stage, learning and honing his skills in travelling repertory companies. In

1998, he played Jack in the Liverpool Everyman Theatre production of *Brothers of the Brush*. Written by the Irish writer Jimmy Murphy, the play is set in 1990s Ireland and revolves around the lives of a small group of house painters working in the black economy. In my role as a supportive wife, I saw the play a number of times. So much so, I knew Tony's part off by heart. During the last performance I fell asleep. There are only so many times one can be enthralled by the same thing. Even the most supportive wife has her limits.

It was fine to be in a theatre with Tony as long as he was on stage. It was a complete nightmare to be in the audience with him, however. Once, while we were in London, a friend gave us tickets for *An Inspector Calls*. The first half of the play was more or less ruined for me by Tony's running commentary on everything from the set to the actors, to the quality of the direction and anything else that crossed his mind. Tony could not whisper, so he was disturbing several rows around us. How we were not asked to leave I do not know. I was glad to get my hands on a glass of wine in the interval. It helped to soothe my murderous thoughts. As the three-minute bell went, Tony decided he had better use the toilet. I grabbed the opportunity to escape from him. During the first half I had spotted where there were some empty seats – and that is where I headed. As I sat down the old lady in the seat next to me said, 'I really don't blame you, dear. What a dreadful man.' I could only agree. I was able to check furtively whether Tony had made his way back to his seat. At the end of the play, when I caught up with him, I claimed I had forgotten where we were sitting. I had my fingers crossed behind my back.

The success of the stage productions in Liverpool and of Prize Night at the Royal Exchange Theatre in Manchester was a factor in encouraging Tony to accept the role of Bottom. The initial rehearsals for *A Midsummer Night's Dream* were held in London. This meant Tony had good theatrical digs – free and comfortable – with his eldest daughter in Downing Street. I was still in Ireland, but it was not long before I had a call from Tony's agent, John Markham. John was becoming increasingly concerned that Tony was finding it hard to cope with the physical demands of rehearsals. He had gone from an excited high to being stressed and miserable. After some discussion, John and I decided that I should travel to London for a few days to keep Tony company and cheer him up before going home. It was always the plan that I would return for the stage run to look after Tony, providing moral support and making sure he was not getting too tired. But then, after I arrived in Leeds for the theatre run, things started to get more complicated.

I have a pacemaker. In fact, I am on my second one, having worn the first one out. My consultant had advised me of two things. One: if I was going to drink wine, it should be red wine in moderation, as it would be better for my heart. I was and continue to be happy to go with this advice. Two: do not get stressed. The second tip has always been the hardest to follow – and never more so than during this production. Tony's self-confidence was being eroded partly by the tiredness caused by a performance each evening and two further afternoon matinees. I was concerned he was beginning to doubt his own skills and abilities. I was upset for him, but not sure what I could do to help.

Tony's distress and my concern to support and protect him led to my stress levels going through the roof, and I collapsed. As I know from previous experiences, landing with a thump on a hard surface really hurts. I have in the past fractured my skull and broken both my legs, at the same time. I was taken by ambulance to hospital, where I had the usual blood tests to make sure I had not had a heart attack. Thankfully the tests were negative, but I didn't feel terribly well.

This was when John Markham decided enough was enough. John contacted the director to let him know he was pulling Tony from the production. I needed to go home and neither Tony nor John was prepared to let me travel or be at home alone. Even though I had some nasty bruises and grazes, I have never been so grateful to have one of my falling-down experiences. The peace and comfort of home was where we wanted to be.

But what I had not factored into my initial concerns about Tony taking on the role of Bottom was the possibility of emotional and mental stress. For some time after we returned home, Tony was angry and tired and felt abused by his recent experience. Each day was a continuous pattern of his rage and frustration – and I was the butt of it all. We had blazing rows as I severely objected to this treatment. It was a horrible time. Everything was my fault, and all the while I was still recovering from my fall. Tony refused to get out of bed until well into the afternoon. I know now depression is another symptom of dementia and staying in bed can be an indication of that. At the time, I simply thought he was being selfish and stupid – which he was, but there was a reason for it.

Looking back, I can see this was the point at which Tony began to lose his resilience; and he would never again do stage work. There was a similar moment when he was still using buses. He loved having a bus pass, as by this stage he could no longer drive and his bus pass was a gateway to some freedom and independence. On one occasion, bundled up against the cold, he could not immediately find his pass when he got on the bus. Losing patience, the bus driver told Tony to go and sit down, but before Tony could reach a seat the irritated driver drove off and he almost fell over. Tony was so shaken he refused to travel on the bus again. Lack of understanding. Thoughtless behaviour. A life undermined.

Eventually, the stress around the production of *A Midsummer Night's Dream* faded enough for life to return to something resembling normal. One of the few pluses of Alzheimer's is that over the course of time he forgot all about it. One of the huge negatives is that you just don't know when the next crisis will occur – and they often came out of left-field. A particularly difficult one occurred when I went to Manchester on one of my twice-yearly pacemaker check-ups. I would usually take the opportunity to spend a few days in Manchester, catching up with family and friends. On the flight home from one trip, it crossed my mind that Tony and I should really make our wills. The morning after returning home, I tried to discuss this with Tony, who seemed not altogether engaged with the conversation. Finally, realising I was getting nowhere fast, I called our solicitor to make an appointment. When I told her what it was for, she seemed surprised, asking if this would be instead of the will Tony had made a few days ago. I had no idea what she was talking about.

Under questioning, Tony revealed that while I was away in Manchester he had made a will. In it, he intended to leave his half of our house to his daughter Cherie. And if I wanted to stay in the house I would have to pay rent to her. I went completely ballistic while he started shouting that it was my own fault, that I should not have left him – and what did I expect? That was when, for the first and only time in our married life, I left him. My bag was still more or less packed from the previous day. Grabbing it and the car key, I walked out. As I drove away, he stood on the doorstep, bellowing at me to never come back. Thank goodness we lived in a secluded spot.

Cursing Tony's behaviour, I went to stay with friends. I did not contact him. After a few days he telephoned me.

'When are you coming home?' he asked, as if nothing had happened.

'I'm not,' was my reply.

Astonished, he said, 'You can't do that. I can't live here on my own. You know I can't. You've got to come home.'

I didn't rush, I stayed away a few more days, but I did go home.

Over time, I became used to this pattern of behaviour. Tony would do something. I would be angry, or fed up. He would carry on as if nothing had happened – and what was I making such a fuss about? As his Alzheimer's progressed, the interval between the deed and the carry-on-as-normal became shorter and shorter. In the end, it was in the space between the next breath. He would look at me, asking, 'What have I done now?' By then I understood and was far more accepting of what was happening. Whilst absolutely craving love, Tony could make himself very difficult to like – let alone love. But love him I did. Despite myself. (I, of course, am perfect!)

Still, at this point in our story, there were relatively long periods of calm when we simply bumbled along in each other's company. We loved taking the dogs to the coast, particularly out of season, when the Atlantic was roaring and crazy. The noise was tremendous and the power of the waves awe-inspiring. We would usually go to Rossnowlagh, where local legend has it Tony Blair learned to swim as a boy. His mother was from Ballyshannon, a small town not far from there.

One summer's day, as we drove along pretty country lanes to the beach, I spotted a man in the hedge. Stopping the car, I got out and walked back to where he was. He had come off his bike and landed in the hedge, where it appeared he was stuck. When we lived in Manchester, I would have thought twice about stopping to help, but in rural Ireland I had no fear. At first, I thought he was unconscious, but quickly realised he was, in fact, dead drunk. I tried to heave the bike out of the way and the man, beginning to come round at the disturbance, started shouting at me. He thought I was trying to steal his bike. My English accent must have surprised him as he stopped trying to fight me. Perhaps he thought he was hallucinating? Hearing me shout, Tony came to help and we untangled the man and his bike from the hedge. He obviously needed to sleep it off on the grassy bank, so we tugged and pulled him into the rescue position, propped his bike up against the hedge and left him to it. On our way back he was gone, we assumed home. A short moment in time, but one Tony always remembered. When conversation became elusive, this was one of his funny stories.

Between Rossnowlagh and Ballyshannon is a hamlet, Creevy Pier. The hotel there has amazing views out across the ocean and serves, in my humble opinion, the best Guinness in Ireland. It is nectar from the gods. Tony and I would often call in there for a drink on the way home. In the winter, it was the perfect place to watch the most amazing sunsets. In the summer, when the evenings were warm and long, we would sit and watch children jumping from the pier into the water. They'd be having such a wonderful time, laughing and egging each other on. It was perfection and remains for me a wonderful, sun-washed memory.

It was on another of our jaunts that we had a dreadful fright. On our way to Carrick-on-Shannon, we were stuck in roadworks in Dowra. Suddenly, the back passenger door of the car was pulled open and someone jumped in behind us. When we first moved to Ireland, we had a visit from the police to discuss our security. Although the Peace Agreement was holding, it was still very new. With this in mind, our first reaction was to look at each other in horror. Then, turning round, we saw an ancient nun sitting on the back seat of our car. As the lights turned to green she urged us forward. I tried to ask her where she was going, but could not make out a word she was saying. Her lack of teeth and thick accent were not conducive to conversation. Eventually, I understood she wanted a lift to a convent in the next town. We drove along in virtual silence, there not being a lot to say. She grabbed my shoulder to indicate we had arrived at her destination and out she jumped. When we arrived in Carrick-on-Shannon, our friends thought we were looking a little pale. We explained what had happened and they started laughing. This nun was well known for jumping into cars. It was a habit of hers to do this when she wanted to get somewhere. The locals were used to her, but we never saw her again. Perhaps she took our virtual silence as an indicator of how unfriendly English people are.

When we made the decision to move to Ireland it was in the full knowledge that at some point we would probably run out of money, yet we did it anyway. It wasn't only about money in the end, but there came a point after about four years in Ireland when Tony and I had to talk about possibly moving back to England. We began to understand that, much as we would want to stay, realistically it would not be possible. My job with the *Irish Times* writing about rural Ireland had come to an end. It had provided us with a regular income – something not too common in the acting profession. That said, Tony was still working fairly regularly in television roles. This income meant we were able to keep putting off a decision. Finally, however, that was no longer possible. Though Tony was still fit enough to be able to work, this would not always be the case. He was in his early seventies. Time and his previously rackety lifestyle would inevitably start catching up with him and it would be easier if he didn't have to travel from Ireland to work.

In addition to this, I had been researching dementia. Although I didn't talk to Tony about it, I was increasingly concerned we might need the support of family and friends if his health seriously declined. I shudder to think of the rows we would have had if I had raised dementia as another reason for going back to England. Running out of money was one thing. Dementia was something else altogether.

The decision to return was made, but after our last house-hunting experience, Tony decided he would stay at home with the dogs and cats while I went to England. Wanting to return to the north-west, but not the same place – in my opinion it is never a good idea to go back – our preferred area was the Upper Calder Valley. I stayed with our friends Steve and Jan, who were going to help me with my search. They have been my friends for over forty years, they know my foibles and, as luck would have it, we found a house on the very first day. A small, mid-terrace former weaver's cottage with a garden. This was the home where Tony would draw his last breath.

Our house in Ireland sold very quickly and we moved to Todmorden in December 2005. This was the first time Tony had seen our new home. He was pleased, as I knew he would be. There had been a fire in the house and although it was sold as 'renovated', we discovered there was a lot to do to make it into the home we wanted. We had to renovate the renovations. As these things do, it took a long time. When Tony died, the only thing left to complete was to replace the back door. Over the course of twelve years, three wooden doors succumbed to winter conditions. Ignoring aesthetics, I finally had to give in and have a composite door made and fitted. I am not sure how far Tony would have approved as he always wanted a wooden door and considered anything else unacceptable. The saving grace is that the door is a pretty shade of green, his favourite colour.

We loved our little house. I quite deliberately set out to make it a safe place for us, as I intuitively understood this was going to be important. I remember coming home one afternoon once to find a strange man in the house. Tony was convinced he knew him. He did not. This man, who turned out to be a stringer for a national tabloid, had turned up on the doorstep and convinced Tony he was an old friend, neglecting to mention he was a journalist. Tony had made him tea and they were sat at the table, chatting away, with Tony, totally unsuspecting, answering his questions. Tony did not understand he was being interviewed. I do not appreciate anyone gaining access to my home by devious means. This man tried to convince me of the same story he had spun for Tony, but as my grandmother would have said, I did not come down with the last shower and the stringer was speedily sent on his way.

For me, this incident was an early indication that Tony was losing his ability to make a quick analysis of a social situation and to behave appropriately. I can imagine the reporter was hail-fellow-well-met when Tony opened the door and that is what Tony would have responded to. He clearly did not stop to consider the man's assertion of knowing him for years. Up to this point, it had not occurred to me that Tony would let a stranger into the house. He was still in the early stages of dementia, but he could be easily confused. I had to make it very clear to him that when I was not there, he was not to let anyone into the house no matter what tale they might tell him. Caring for someone with dementia is a constant readjustment to changing circumstances and unpredictable needs. Interestingly, from the point of view of the development of his Alzheimer's, Tony could not understand my reaction to the reporter. He thought I was being rude. I was, but I was also being protective. It was disturbing to think of who else he might have let in. The journalist was bad enough, but heavens above, alternative scenarios were much more concerning.

In an effort to get involved in the community when we returned to England, Tony and I re-joined the Labour Party. Some of the people we met at the local branch have remained our friends ever since. Tony still had strong opinions and was happy to be involved in campaigns. No one ever doubted his socialist credentials. It was mine that came under scrutiny, even though we were married. Some members of the Party who styled themselves as hard left appeared to blame me for those of Tony Blair's policies they did not agree with. It did not seem to matter to them that the Prime Minister did not consult me, not even once, on any political decisions. It was a good stick to beat me with, particularly during the 2010 General Election when I was the Labour candidate for the Calder Valley. It was also a good excuse for them not to campaign. I came second in the election, so not a complete wipe-out, despite their best efforts. This was the point at which Tony became utterly disenchanted with the Labour Party. His position was always that the Party is bigger than any individual and, as members, it is important to get behind the selected candidate; you do not actually have to like them. (Even so, if he had not already been a life member by then, Tony would have left the Party when Jeremy Corbyn was elected leader.) I knew my political opponents were generating rumours and false stories about us both, but more specifically about me. With the benefit of hindsight, I can see they made me out to be much more interesting than I actually am. Some sort of bonus, I suppose. One of the rumours concerned our move to Ireland. Apparently we had been ordered out of the country by Tony Blair, who thought my Tony a blot on the landscape of his government. Can you imagine? Worse, the person who repeated the story to me absolutely believed it. Poor old Ireland. Not quite Devil's Island, but ... !

Living through Tony's dementia was tough, and as a result specific dates and times become easily blurred in my head.

But I do know it was sometime during the summer of 2010 when Tony made his bombshell announcement.

We were sitting in the garden on our favourite bench by the pond. It is a good place to admire the dragonflies and play 'Spot the Frog'. Unusually, when he started talking to me he did not look at me. He was gazing straight ahead. He was not speaking very clearly, so I had to ask him to repeat himself. Turning towards me, he shouted, 'I have to stop working. I cannot be an actor. My memory isn't good enough anymore.' No wonder he shouted. I can only imagine what it cost him to articulate this thought. I tried to take his hand, but he shook me off.

One of the chief certainties of our life together had always been that Tony was an actor. His announcement was like someone loosening the keystone in an arch. Things could and probably would come tumbling down, but who could know when? I felt myself becoming tearful. We sat in silence for a few minutes. Then, although he was no longer shouting, Tony became angry. He insisted no one was to know of his decision, particularly his agent. I was the only person who needed to know. We sat for a few more minutes until, blowing my nose, I went into the house to make a pot of tea. An utterly banal reaction, I know, but it was the only thing I could think to do.

We never spoke of this conversation again. Tony would still talk about his acting career, the things he had done and the people he had met. His failing memory was never mentioned. If anyone asked about future acting roles, he would laughingly dismiss the question with an 'I'm too old for all of that now.'

So, we had begun the dementia game. It was called 'Cover Up'. Tony's decision was in no way an acceptance on his part that he had dementia. As I've explained, he would never admit that. Eventually, he would begin to come to terms with having Alzheimer's, but he would not be demented. In a tough negotiating situation, sometimes semantics is all. Alzheimer's, in his mind, had nothing to connect it with dementia.

I remember being invited to a meeting in London organised by the Alzheimer's Society. It was an afternoon event and a couple of the charity's ambassadors were talking about their experiences of family members with dementia. At the end there was a short Q&A session. One man raised this same issue. Why did the disease have to be named dementia, with all the negative and hopeless connotations of that word? 'Demented' brings to mind Lear being lashed by the storm as he carries Cordelia's lifeless body. The man posing the question did not want to be demented any more than Tony did. Any more than any human would. But there was no answer for him. I know changing the name of the disease does not change the reality of it. It would perhaps, though, make it slightly more bearable and slightly less fearsome.

Having made the decision to retire, it was almost as if Tony now gave himself permission to give in to dementia. There was increasing forgetfulness and confusion, but he was still able to function at a reasonably normal level – whatever 'normal' is. What was getting ever more difficult to cope with were his temper and mood swings. One moment he would be fine, the next he was raging about something insignificant. Or perhaps something that I considered insignificant.

I arranged a GP appointment for Tony. Of course, I went with him. I needed to explain my concerns. At this stage in his dementia, Tony was lucid more often than not; he was an actor and still perfectly capable of assuming a plausible demeanour. Talking to the doctor, he was calm and collected – with really no idea what I was going on about. I had to be very persuasive and very insistent for the doctor to refer Tony for a brain scan. The ace up my sleeve was the tentative diagnosis by the Irish psychologist.

Tony refused point-blank to go to the first appointment for a scan. Nothing I said would convince him to change his mind. He was scared and I could not get past that. I telephoned and cancelled the appointment, but I also made another one. This time, I enlisted the help of Cherie. We devised a plan. We would both talk to him, but under no circumstances would we mention Alzheimer's, and least of all dementia. We would discuss what a pain it was getting old and how forgetting things was such a nuisance. If he had the scan, the doctor would then be able to prescribe something that might help. It was an entirely reasonable plan, with the added advantage that it played into Tony's hypochondria and his enjoyment of pill regimes. Years ago, the *Guardian* newspaper used to run a short feature in their Saturday magazine about bizarre and interesting diseases. Without fail, Tony would decide it was the featured disease, whatever it was, that had been causing him problems all these years. He was not joking. I started hiding the magazine.

At the second time of trying, Tony had his brain scan. When we went back to the GP surgery for the results, it was not our doctor we saw but a psychologist. The scan revealed Tony had Alzheimer's. Weirdly, though, the psychologist was insistent there was nothing wrong with Tony, despite the evidence. As we sat in her office, Tony was entirely lucid and it became clear this woman considered *me* to be the one with issues. I tried to explain again about my concerns, but she was not listening, preferring instead to chat to Tony. To my complete frustration, she was convinced by his performance. She was also star struck. At the end of our appointment, she simply said to me, 'Yes, we have a diagnosis, but I'm not sure it's right – take him home and get on with it.' No advice. No offer of support. Not even any suggestion where I might begin to find any of the above.

So, once again, we came home from seeing a psychologist without any clear information about what to do next. To be fair, the doctor in Ireland had been honest and said he could not be certain of a diagnosis. At the time, given the uncertainty I too felt about Tony's behaviour, this seemed fine. Things were not getting any worse and in fact remained stable for a couple of years. However, back in England, and despite having the results of Tony's brain scan, the second psychologist was dismissive of clear evidence. This was one of my first lessons in what seemed to be the inadequacy of the medical profession when it came to the treatment and understanding of dementia and of its ramifications for sufferer and carer alike.

As I'd anticipated, the lucid man in the doctor's office was unable to maintain that level of performance at home. I could see Tony's levels of frustration and distress increasing as the limiting effects of dementia also increased. For a lot of the time, our life together continued much as it always had, but now with the ever-present threat of furious outbursts from Tony.

It was not many weeks before we were back in the doctor's office and this time I had a more sympathetic hearing. The GP was as surprised as I was by the psychologist's rejection of the scan evidence. I had done some research and come across a drug called Aricept. I do not know the current situation, but certainly back then the drug was not routinely prescribed. After some discussion, our GP thought it was worth trying. The drug works by increasing the levels and activity of acetylcholine, a chemical messenger in the brain which may help to alleviate the symptoms of Alzheimer's disease. At the time, I was not much concerned about how the drug worked; I simply wanted it to work – and it certainly helped Tony for quite some time and, by default, me. One of the interesting facts I did discover is that different health authorities have varying attitudes towards prescribing Aricept. The strength of Tony's dosage increased over time until he reached the maximum allowed under our local health authority. Other authorities would have allowed his dosage to increase further, but I was unable to find out the reason for these varying policy decisions.

Tony and I always enjoyed our expeditions and the effect of Aricept made them easier. We enjoyed exploring and pottering around, taking in new surroundings. One of our expeditions took us to Strasbourg on an organised coach trip with our friends Mike and Jennifer. None of us was particularly good at being organised and shepherded about by others, so we would break off and do our own thing; though, of course, we were fully signed up when it came to the trip to the European Parliament.

As we queued to go into the public gallery of the parliamentary chamber, Tony decided it would be a good idea to use the lavatory first. A sensible decision, given how he was becoming increasingly anxious about wetting himself. I offered to go with him and help him find his way back, but unintentionally embarrassed him by suggesting this while we were stood in the queue. His response was to be loudly sarcastic, asking if I thought he was totally stupid. As people turned to look, I wanted the ground to swallow me up. Tony went off one way and I went the other, into the gallery. What I should have done was wait for him.

As we filed in, I knew there was little point in trying to save Tony a seat next to me. He would have to find a place at the end of a row. I kept a lookout for him, but it was a bit difficult as the gallery was rather cramped and there were a lot of people in there. At one point, I stood up to try to see him, before deciding it might be a good idea to go and find him. Shuffling along the row, past everyone, I managed to work my way out and went straight to the men's loo. There was no sign of Tony outside. Taking a deep breath – how many social protocols was I breaking here? – I pushed open the door and went in to look for him. I knew he was unlikely to be in there after all this time, but I needed to make sure he hadn't collapsed in one of the cubicles. He wasn't there either.

I had no idea where to start looking next. I walked along the corridor, checking everywhere I could. I then went down to the next level to search for him. I could hear my heart starting to thump in my ears. I left the building to see if he had gone outside for a crafty cigarette – still no sign of him. I went back to the gallery and, managing to catch Mike's eye, I indicated I needed him and Jennifer to come out into the corridor. That was when the three of us became seriously worried for Tony's safety. Jennifer, who is eminently sensible, decided we had to inform security and get their help in locating Tony. But where were they? We went downstairs and by a stroke of luck bumped into Linda McAvan, our local

MEP. She immediately contacted security and the hunt for Tony was on. He could not be found. Was it possible he had gone back to the coach? I shook my head, confident he would not have been able to make his way back there on his own.

When we finally decided to check the coach, there was Tony stretched out, fast asleep on the back seat. I could not believe he had found the coach park, let alone the right coach. I was livid with him for frightening me like that. Before I could do or say anything, Jennifer put her hand on my shoulder and said, 'Please don't kill him, Steph.'

It was at moments like this when the dementia seemed to fall away and Tony was suddenly able to do something I'd believed was now totally beyond him, giving me false hope. Intellectually, I knew he would never get better, but emotionally I was still grasping at straws. To be honest, right to the end those straws were still proving elusive.

Finding him was not, however, the end of the Strasbourg incident. The next time Tony and I visited Cherie, she asked me about it. How on earth did she know? It turns out Kathryn Blair's boyfriend, James, was working in the European Parliament at the time. The news that Tony Blair's father-in-law was lost soon spread around the building. James told Kathryn, who then told her mother, who in turn asked me about it. There was no question of covering our tracks. That family have a network the Tudor spymaster Robert Cecil would have been proud of!

5.

Breaking point

Tony's Alzheimer's played out in the small adjustments, the sometimes virtually imperceptible changes. Things such as one day struggling to get his socks on, or being unable to fasten the buttons on his shirt when the day before there had been no problem. It was one of the first signs of diminishing hand–eye co-ordination, but for a long time Tony was able to dress himself if I lay his clothes out on the bed in the right order for him to put them on. The only problems would be if he pushed the pile of clothes to one side, so he could sit on the bed. That would lead to confusion and questions such as 'Are you sure my vest goes over my shirt?' He would sometimes try to hand me something for me to put on him, but I would not help when I knew he was capable of doing something for himself. It may sound brutal, but tough love was the only way for him to stay functioning at even the most basic level. A skill lost was a skill gone for ever and the aim was to hang on to them for as long as possible.

So, we did not tumble headlong into catastrophe. Tony's deterioration was initially a much more gradual decline. At first, I was foolishly hopeful his dementia wouldn't prove to be any big deal. And, essentially, our lives would bumble along on a fairly contented plateau – but then out of the blue there would be an event that we would fall through until we reached the next plateau. Things would then even out for a while again. Tony's rage and frustration would calm down, but some part of his personality and skill set would always disappear – lost for ever. As a carer, this really is tough. It means watching someone disintegrate in front of you. Horrible, horrible – but then you have to learn quickly to make the best of, and live with, what's left.

Other people who knew him would notice the changes in him and I would see they were right. Tony's behaviour could occasionally be unexpected, but nothing I couldn't deal with. I'd had plenty of training beforehand in dealing with Tony's eccentricities, so dementia wasn't really throwing up any surprises at this point. He could inflict embarrassment and I was used to that, but there was one time when he was utterly excruciating and even I blanched. We were in Berlin with our Irish friends Breda and Tommy and travelling on a busy tram between the railway station and the Brandenburg Gate. Tony and I were sat together, looking out of the window, when he suddenly said, 'You know something, I think we did them a favour bombing the shit out of them during the war. Look at how fantastic the city is now.'

'Will you please shut up?'

'What's your problem? None of them speak any English.'

Then a German voice carried across the tram: 'Some of us do.' I understood what no one else on the tram did – it was his dementia and increasing loss of social inhibition making him behave in this way. Even so, I couldn't wait to get off the tram, so I could berate him without an audience.

Later the same day, we went to the Reichstag, the parliament building, to see the glass dome designed by English architect Norman Foster. Everything was fine until we began our descent of the spiralling ramps. They are beautiful, open and light, but I was overwhelmed by vertigo and felt a desperate need to lie flat on the ground. Really, I should have had more sense and simply admired the dome from the outside at ground level, as this was not the first time I had experienced this problem.

I don't know what triggered Tony's irritation, but he was clearly cross, wanting to know why I was being so stupid and drawing all this attention to myself. He was probably getting tired and in need of cake. As a former alcoholic, he had a very sweet tooth; sugar was essential to his good mood. He walked off ahead, occasionally turning round to tell me to hurry up, leaving Tommy and Breda to help and support me getting down the ramps. I could not understand why he was being so horrible – and in public too. My children knew they might sometimes get away with misbehaving at home, but outside the house such misdemeanours carried heavy penalties. Now, I understand that loss of empathy is yet another symptom of dementia.

*

Upsetting though this incident was, it was nothing like what was to come. I do wonder if Alzheimer's and Asperger's share similar symptoms – the need for routines to provide security in an increasingly confusing world. Did Tony's own anxieties overwhelm any empathy he had? I was the security blanket to his Charlie Brown and no weakness of mine could be allowed to threaten that. I had to develop strategies to help cope with my own anger when Tony was this unpleasant and difficult. One of them was thinking in terms of 'my Tony', the man I married, and Tony the person I was living with now – the stranger I was sharing my life with. My Tony would not have behaved as Tony did at the Reichstag. My Tony would have been concerned about my fear and wanted to help.

It was all very well me having strategies, but they could conflict with the reality I was dealing with. I am not a saint and it is extremely unlikely, given my personality, I will ever become one. Exasperation and sympathy were emotions that frequently battled within me; I would often go through a short-lived explosion, then calm down and deal with it. I was determined to hold our lives together, dealing with each day, hour and incident as it happened – for good, or bad. Attempting to be a 'good wife' or a 'good carer', forever patient and understanding, would have pushed me over the edge.

Ascribing all of Tony's behavioural issues to dementia was easy if you were not living with him. He could be crafty and

I sometimes wouldn't know if he was aware of what he was doing. Sometimes I would give him the benefit of the doubt, sometimes I wouldn't and a row would ensue.

When we first got together, Tony's theatrical rages used to unnerve me. A raised voice capable of booming around a theatre was not pleasant in the close confines of a kitchen. But then I got wise. He thought the loudest voice would win the day. It did for a while until I deployed my own tactics. My grandmother always claimed I had a tongue like a box of knives and in a row I could usually best Tony. 'You think you're so clever,' he would yell. 'That's because I am,' would be my response. That would usually make him laugh and the row would be over, but as dementia claimed him he could not defend himself in this sort of verbal sparring. His lexicon was diminishing and his brain was not working fast enough – it was a most unequal fight. To bring the argument to an end, I would announce I was going to make a pot of tea – and would he like some biscuits to go with it? That would usually disarm him and he would settle into his favourite armchair, waiting to be looked after. Sometimes, though, he wanted to sulk and would refuse the tea and biscuits to punish me, but the row was nevertheless over.

One of the ways the cruelty of this disease manifested itself was by gradually taking away Tony's ability to communicate. It wasn't just a question of losing words: he lost the ability to hold conversations as he couldn't remember what had just been said. It would be a devastating experience for anyone, but perhaps more so for an actor – the art of communication was a vital part of who he was. I am grateful dementia never quite won that battle. Up until a few hours before he died, he was still trying to talk and make me and the district nurses laugh. Having told his stories so many times, he could still remember them – usually the most outrageous ones. He would tell his stories as a way of continuing to relate to people.

Of course, not being able to talk to me without struggling for lost words frustrated him. I couldn't do right for doing wrong. If I suggested any words, that made him feel patronised. If I remained silent, waiting for him to tell me himself, then I was being unhelpful.

'You know the thing that you put on the whatsit to make it work – what's it called?'

'Tell me what you use it for and I'll try to help.'

Gesticulations like some manic game of Charades would follow as he reached desperately for the word. I was quite good at guessing, but sometimes I failed and I began to realise how tiring Tony's frustration was for me. When he was first diagnosed, I believed I was Superwoman, and able to cope on my own with Tony's dementia. Really, what was there to worry about? He seemed fine back in those days, when all I had to live with was his fairly mild confusion. Crikey, how wrong can you be? It is only when you live with someone who has the disease you realise how utterly exhausting it is.

When Tony was first diagnosed, he was assigned a social worker to help us and organise support for us. Unfortunately,

Tony had a low opinion of social workers and refused to treat them with respect. One visit and they were gone, never to return, unable to deal with his rude and overbearing behaviour, which he would adopt especially for them. In the end, I would prefer not sit in on these visits. I couldn't bear the tension and my desire to tell Tony to pack it in – which is what he wanted, so he could start an argument with me as well as the social worker. Then Lydia walked into our lives in a flurry of gorgeous red hair and a very nice handbag. Tony was stunned, which was a good start. The three of us sat round the table and Tony began his routine. He had barely started before Lydia intervened and told him his behaviour was not acceptable, it was to stop and he was to answer her questions as best he could.

There had been suggestions from other professionals that Tony might go to a day centre a couple of days a week, so he could experience the company of different people and I could have a break from caring for him. His refusal was adamant. He didn't want to spend the day with a load of old people with whom he would have nothing in common – and, anyway, why did I need a rest, because he didn't need looking after? I have no idea how she did it – an amazing combination of cunning and guile, impressive to watch – but Lydia persuaded Tony the day centre was a good idea. As soon as she got back to the office, she made the arrangements. For the first time, I felt not so much that someone was on my side, but that someone was determined to support me in the day-to-day care for Tony. It was a huge relief.

However, Tony's agreeing to the day centre was one thing. Getting him to leave the house when the bus arrived was quite another. The first time the driver came for him, Tony refused to go, though he did go the second time. The three of us – Cherie, Lydia and me – all exerted some pretty lethal pressure. Tony always caved in to women; he claimed it started with his mother. It was one of the great problems or pleasures of his life, depending on how you want to look at it.

I often spent those two days a week in our garden, which was a nightmare when we first moved in. We had to remove three tons of household rubbish, ten conifers and twenty-eight plastic garden gnomes and their specially constructed home. I was keen to create a space where Tony and I could sit in the summer surrounded by pleasant scents and colours that would remind him of his childhood and the garden he had made for his mother. Good memories became incredibly important to him. They were a safe place to retreat to when needed and were increasingly more vivid and certain than his new reality.

I joined the RHS and the National Trust, and we would go on days out to look at the gardens and have lunch – another thing Tony always enjoyed and which also helped to maintain his social skills. We must have looked like Darby and Joan as he held on to my arm and we wandered happily along the pathways between beautiful flower beds. Garden benches are a good, calm place to just sit and be. Even when we were broke and on an alleged economy drive, we tended to come back with a plant from wherever we had visited. Once they were planted, it was a good way of jogging Tony's memory, reminding him of our day out. I knew he probably couldn't remember the details, but what he could do was recall the feeling of pleasure he would have felt. He would always remark how much he enjoyed our jaunts.

We would have perfectly amiable and happy days, but Tony's dementia was increasingly progressing from forgetfulness and confusion to rage and frustration. Very negative emotions were now tormenting him. Taking him out helped to soothe him, but we couldn't go out every day. For one thing, he would have found it too exhausting. Having smoked since he was eleven, nicotine consumption was catching up with his heart and lungs. I was asked many times why I didn't try to make him put a stop to his smoking, but what would have been the point? He was old, the damage had been done and there was no longer any good reason for him to stop. It would have only made him miserable.

It was an expensive habit, but Cherie would bring back cartons of duty-free cigarettes for him when she went on her travels. In the end, I had to ask her to give them to me rather than her dad, as Tony believed it was his purpose in life to work his way through them all as quickly as possible. This reached the pinnacle of daftness when on one occasion

I found him with a lit cigarette in each hand. I began hiding his tobacco stash, but despite his dementia he would always discover the hiding place. Eventually, I realised secreting them in plain sight was the most effective. Smoking was part of who he was and was something he could hold on to. In a funny kind of way, it gave meaning to his life. When other bits of his personality were falling away and disappearing, smoking didn't for a long time.

People who smoke claim it calms them down: they will need a cigarette if they're feeling stressed or anxious. Interestingly, it no longer had this effect on Tony. He smoked because he had always smoked and it was something he remembered how to do. I'm not sure how much, in the end, he really enjoyed cigarettes and certainly for several months before he died he'd stopped smoking altogether – because he'd forgotten he was a smoker. And I failed to remind him.

There were times when I really wished the nicotine would soothe him – particularly when he was aggressive, or frustrated. He went through an extended middle period when his Alzheimer's had progressed from the early stages of confusion and forgetfulness, but before the disease had overtaken him and he became much more passive. It is this middle stage that is the most difficult, most brutal and most destructive for both the sufferer and those close to them.

Tony was no longer sleeping well at night. He was spending a lot of time asleep in the day, so of course he wasn't tired when we went to bed at night. He didn't lie quietly in bed, waiting to go back to sleep; he would be up and down to the bathroom, turning on the bedroom light and generally being a complete nuisance. I was then in my fifties with my days of small children and broken nights at least twenty years behind me. If lack of sleep had been tough then, in middle age it was murder. When I could no longer cope, Lydia suggested Tony go into respite care for a week, so I could have a complete rest.

For me, it was a brilliant idea. Tony, on the other hand, was not impressed. He kept asking me over and over again what I intended to do during this time, all the while becoming more and more convinced that I intended to go away with another man. In reality, chance would have been a fine thing; and, more crucially, I was far too exhausted to think about, let alone get involved with, anything as time-consuming and demanding as an affair. My only fantasy was to be in bed alone and enjoy hours of unbroken sleep. Yet Tony became fixated on my 'unfaithful' behaviour, telling anyone, including complete strangers, about it. Looking back, I can see this was probably more fear than jealousy. I was the constant support in his life – whatever else was going on, he still recognised how much he needed me and was afraid of me disappearing. Perversely, I think he was also angry about this neediness. He was a proud man.

Several times, I wavered in my resolve to send Tony into respite care, but logically I knew I could not continue without a break from this level of responsibility. I was by this point taking citalopram, an antidepressant, on the basis that it provided me with a vital crutch, helping me to achieve what Tony and I both wanted: for him to live at home. I was desperately tired and I'm hopeless when tired. I get weepy and bad tempered, and it is a fact that the whole world is against me – or so it feels. Although friends were shocked, some of them believing this was a step too far and that if I needed drugs to cope then Tony should be *in* a home rather than *at* home, the citalopram helped to keep me on a more even keel. Problems remained, but they did not seem so completely insurmountable.

However, the drugs could not help with or soothe everything. One morning, Tony had come into my work room to chat and question me, once again, about what I intended to do with my time while he was in respite care. Eventually, as I had things to do, I suggested to him that he should have a shower and get dressed. He left begrudgingly. While I fired up the computer, I had my back to the door and didn't hear Tony re-enter the room. He came up behind me and smacked me hard around the back of my head. I hadn't seen or heard him approach, and he caught me entirely by surprise. The force of the blow hurt my eyes and I bit my tongue hard. There was blood pouring out of my mouth, but more than anything I was completely shocked.

I sat there for a moment and by the time I'd stood up, Tony had locked himself in the bathroom and was shouting at me through the door that he hadn't hit me. He wouldn't let me in the bathroom, so I couldn't get a towel for my face and I had to rummage about in the dirty washing basket for a relatively clean T-shirt to mop up the blood. Tony's incessant and repetitive questions and ridiculous accusations were one thing, but now things really had gone too far and I could not and did not want to cope with Tony's behaviour anymore. I phoned the doctors' surgery, who told me to come in immediately. Listening to me as I explained what had happened, my GP suggested that, for my own safety, Tony would have to be sectioned. I was upset, but knew there was no other option. I had done everything I could to look after Tony and yet it had still come to this.

After the doctor had checked me over and given me a prescription for my sore tongue and aching head, I went home. She wasn't sure that was a good idea, but I knew Tony's behaviour patterns. I knew that after the storm of fury, he would be subdued and wanting everything to be all right again. I kept a low profile until the late afternoon, when the doctor arrived with a policeman and a consultant psychiatrist. As soon as Tony realised who they were and the purpose of their visit, his anger and lack of self-control immediately bubbled over again. He began to try to make them leave the house, displaying exactly the behaviour they were concerned about. He would not co-operate when the doctor tried to talk to him or ask him questions. I was asked to go and pack a small bag for Tony whilst the others attempted to calm him and deal with his rage. I cannot remember how he was persuaded to leave the house, but I seem to remember he trusted the policeman more than the doctors and agreed to go with him in his car to the hospital. Perhaps he hoped the policeman would protect him from these people who wanted to take him away to somewhere he didn't know and was far from happy to go to.

I stood at the door as Tony left with the policeman, who helped him down the steps. Tony looked at me and in that moment I could see he hated me. He really believed I was the enemy, but what was I to do? I could not believe what was happening to us. I had to have time and space to figure out not only if I could go on caring for Tony, but more importantly if I still wanted to. Was I a victim of domestic violence or his dementia, or possibly both? Would I ever be able to trust him again? But these were questions for consideration in a few days' time. At that moment my misery was so overwhelming I could taste it.

After the telephone call from the psychiatric unit, telling me Tony had arrived and they were settling him in, I went to bed, overcome with the dead weight of exhaustion, distress and anger. I remember Tony Blair saying to me once that he would believe anything he heard about my Tony other than that he had hit a woman, yet he had done it to me. My hurt was emotional as well as physical. I slept solidly for ten hours, but didn't really feel any better when I woke up. I have a good support network of friends, but I didn't want to talk to anyone about what had happened, so I went for a long walk across the hills with my dogs in the hope that fresh air would soothe my wounded spirits. In the wide-open and deserted space, I stood on a rock and roared into the wind with the dogs standing guard next to me, unsure of what was happening. I gave myself a sore throat, but it eased my emotional pain.

Returning home, I telephoned the hospital and was told Tony was now calm but not getting out of bed – his go-to place when he wanted to shut out the world. He remained adamant he had not hit me and I was lying if I said he had. I was told it was better for me not to speak to him for a few days, so he would settle and forget what had happened and be relieved to hear from me. I, of course, had my own issues to deal with, including shame. Shame that Tony had been sectioned. I know it was totally irrational to feel like that, but I did. I was also shamed by the fact he had hit me. That did not happen to the kind of tough-minded and intelligent woman I believed myself to be. My self-respect had also taken a hit. When I was in town or in the supermarket, I was convinced that people would be able to tell from my demeanour what had happened.

I felt further undermined when some of Tony's family were angry about my decision to have him sectioned. They may have understood that this was a reasonable reaction to what had happened, but at that time they had very little understanding of the day-to-day reality of living with his illness. Speaking to him on the phone, when he could be entirely lucid for the duration of the call, was no substitute for the lived experience. I stopped answering the phone and made the decision to hide from the world. And I did – except from my close friend Chris, who took it upon herself to feed me every evening, insisting I go to hers, which meant I had no choice but to leave the house.

After almost a week, I went to visit Tony and true to the pattern that had developed over the preceding months, he had completely forgotten about the crisis. Looking at him, I saw a confused, skinny old man who had no idea what was happening to him. His vulnerability was heart-breaking. He was calm and pleased to see me, wanting to know when I was going to take him home. I said it was probably better for him to remain where he was until various tests had been completed. He accepted this, although every time I visited he would ask that same question; but I still had to think through and honestly address some serious issues. Would Tony be better off in a nursing home? Was his care something for professionals to handle, rather than me making it up as I went along and hoping for the best? Did I want him to come home and would I be able to cope if he did? Having survived a violent childhood, should I risk any return to that space? My head was a mess.

I found it really hard to work out. I was furious with Tony for behaving in the way he had, but I was also really angry with a system that had failed me as well as him. The drug he was taking, Aricept, had ceased to have any palliative effect some months earlier and I was once again plunged into the struggle for pharmaceutical support. The NHS Choices website had stated: 'If at any time it appears Aricept has become unsuitable, it is important the prescriber is contacted immediately.' My local health practice was clearly unaware of these guidelines, because I was unable to make clear or convince them of the need for Tony's prescription to be changed. I was told nothing else was available, but I had read about a drug called memantine which can potentially be useful when Aricept no longer is. It is a drug that can be effective for behavioural and psychological symptoms associated with Alzheimer's disease.

It was only after this huge crisis, with Tony ending up on a locked psychiatric ward, that further help became available. During the second and final week of his stay on the ward, Cherie came up from London to join me when the discussion with a consultant psychiatrist about her dad's future took place. I had decided it would be sensible for me to wait for this meeting before I finally made up my mind about whether Tony should come home.

The psychiatrist told us that Tony had been prescribed memantine whilst he was on the ward and she wanted him to continue on it as the drug clearly had a calming effect on him. Given that this was exactly what I had been campaigning for – and for many months – I have no idea why I felt so angry when I heard this. Why is dementia care always about crisis management? Why had no one listened to me? I was the person who looked after him 24/7, so why was my experience not relevant? This whole horrible incident might well have been avoided if Tony had been on the right medication. Was it really the case I had to be injured before anyone listened? To answer my own question – yes, it was the case. In reality, it wasn't just a question of whether I could rely on Tony not being physically violent again, but would I also be able to rely on the medical and caring professions for continuing support following his hospitalisation?

As the discussion went on, it became clear I would be offered a lot of support should I decide that Tony could come home. It was also clear the decision was entirely mine. I was the one who would be looking after him. We can never know the answers, never predict outcomes, especially concerning someone who has dementia – and, in the end, the only thing I did know was I wasn't ready to give up on him yet. When he came out of hospital, Tony went into respite care, so I got my week off in the end, but it had been a hard road to get there. It had been the worst of times. Looking back now, I know I made the right decision, no matter how tough it became. In the end, I did keep my promise – he would stay with me – but I also benefited from the decision as I needed him, too.

When I brought Tony home, he was relieved and happy to be back. The dogs were thrilled to see him, making a huge fuss, and he was pleased to see them. The soothing, unconditional and undemanding affection of pets is a great help to people with dementia. Their familiarity helped settle him back into our home. But it was far from plain sailing, and we were still working through a difficult time as Tony's frustration and confusion about what Alzheimer's was doing to him would continue to spill over. He didn't understand what was happening to him, but he did know it wasn't good. Memantine helped and he started going again to the day centre twice a week, so mostly life was manageable, as I now had the time to draw breath and break out of the dementia bubble occasionally.

I put some new strategies in place, including not walking down the stairs in front of him. The injuries from being pushed would have been quite nasty. I was also more ready to confront him when he was being particularly unpleasant, or unreasonable rather, than always hoping to soothe him. As I've said, given my personality, sainthood is beyond my reach and I knew trying to be forever patient and understanding would push me over the edge – whilst still knowing that possessing a good dose of strength and patience was the only way to cope.

This latest experience made me finally confront the issue I had been avoiding: that Tony and I only had limited time left in which we could still enjoy life together. I needed good and happy memories to hold on to and keep for ever. We made a bucket list and that summer we went to Languedoc. It was somewhere that Tony, with his interest in the Knights Templar, had wanted to go for ages. I thought it was an awfully long way, particularly given that he could no longer fly. Airports had become one of the more testing levels of purgatory. Busy, crowded and generally not very nice, the chances of losing Tony rose exponentially in them, particularly if he couldn't see where I was and wandered off to look for me. The choice was simple: give up flying or buy a set of handcuffs. My pacemaker also meant that going through security could be an ordeal as I couldn't keep an eye on Tony. Invariably, he would forget something metal in his pocket and he would be taken to one side. Then, not being able to understand what he was being asked, he would go into panic mode.

The worst time happened when we were returning home from France and I had some marsh salt from Gironde in my hand luggage. I was being patted down and trying frantically to watch out for Tony when I was approached by a policeman who wanted to know about the white granular stuff in my bag. I told him it was salt.

'Nonetheless, madam, you need to accompany me while we have a look at it,' he said.

Protesting that now really wasn't a good moment, I was taken by the elbow and led to the other side of security where my bag was waiting for me. I tried to tell them I needed to get Tony first and then I would be more than happy to run through their routine. They got very cross with me and threatened to take me into a side room while the 'substance' was checked. By then it felt as if everyone in the airport was watching. I was half dead with embarrassment, yet desperate to spot Tony. Fortunately, a kindly woman understood the situation and brought Tony over.

The first thing he said was, 'What are they doing with your salt?'

'Testing it for drugs.'

He thought this highly amusing given my puritanical attitude to drugs. His laughing at me did not help. This nerve-shredding experience was the last time I ever took Tony through an airport.

So this resulted in Hobson's choice: either I drove to Languedoc or we didn't go. From Todmorden, where we lived, to Arques where we'd rented a gîte is a journey of 1,006.5 miles as the crow flies, without including any detours for wee stops or meals. On the upside, at least I would know where Tony was, I was in charge of our passports and we didn't have to go individually through security. We set off in the middle of August, the car stuffed with all the paraphernalia Tony believed he couldn't live without and with Millie, our Springer Spaniel, stretched out on the back seat. We completed the journey over several days and as we passed around Carcassonne I knew we had come a long way when I saw motorway signs for Barcelona.

Our gîte was only small yet was sufficient for us and opened on to a sun-drenched courtyard. Perfect for enjoying late-afternoon sun with a glass of chilled wine in hand and a good book to read. There were obviously difficult moments, when the strangeness of the place or tiredness got to Tony – he was by then struggling to understand the nuances of English, let alone French. Sometimes he couldn't remember where he was and the answer was to sit for a while, have a cup of coffee or something else to drink and give him time to get back into his head. That said, it was a wonderful holiday and one Tony remembered for a long time.

We were there to look at castles and we were certainly spoiled for choice. It seemed as if there was one perched on top of every inaccessible mountain. Of course I exaggerate, but I couldn't work out how they managed to ferry building materials up there; and the novels Tony had been reading concerned knights of old, their daring deeds and that sort of thing, rather than the nitty-gritty of the ordinary stuff. I thought perhaps it might be another case of Noah's Ark, as given what we are told about Noah, it would seem unlikely he was the one who drew up the spreadsheets, organised the construction and work force and finally the animals going in two by two. I feel Mrs Noah has to be the unsung hero of that story. I tried to impress Tony with this theory, but failed miserably. I only confused him by talking about the Ark as he thought I was talking about the Ark of the Covenant.

The castle Tony was most keen to see was Montségur. It was after lunch and a hot afternoon when we drove into the car park at the bottom of the mountain. Tony looked up at the castle, enquired if there was a funicular operating and when I said no he refused to do the climb. That wasn't an unreasonable decision, but I had driven all the way from West Yorkshire specifically for this moment. I looked at him, debating how well the people in cars nearby might understand English before I gave him the benefit of my opinions – and then decided against this course of action. I settled Tony into a chair, made sure he had his hat on and plenty of water to drink, and left him to read about the castle while Millie and I set off to look at it.

It was something of a strenuous climb, particularly as I was wearing a short skirt and open-toed sandals. A National Trust property, with neatly laid steps and paths, it was not. Reaching the top, I sat on a rock with my back against the castle wall, finding peace and awe in the magnificence of the countryside laid out below me. The journey down was much easier than the journey up and I found Tony, who had somehow invented his own version of Franglais, chatting away to a couple who had placed their chairs next to him. They seemed to be getting on famously. It is one of the strange, unexpected things about dementia: I have no idea of the how and why, but there would be a sudden burst of lucidity and I would have 'my' Tony back, even if only for a few moments. I had taken lots of photographs to show him and we set off again to find a bar and beer so he could look at them. I never knew how keenly or not Tony felt the loss of not being able to do these things himself, but he seemed content to listen to my stories and look at the photographs I'd taken. Increasingly his life was being lived vicariously through mine.

There was a bar just around the corner from where we were staying and on our last night we went there for a drink with Sandra, the gîte owner. The owner of the bar was young, gorgeous and achingly cool – as was the music he played. I can't remember at what point everyone in the bar decided to dance. Piling out of the door, as the bar was too small, a street party started. At first everyone was happy dancing to jazz until Sandra and I decided some ABBA was called for. Specifically, 'Dancing Queen'. The bar owner, whose name I don't recall, was horrified and simply pushed the laptop across the bar and said, 'Go ahead.' That was when the party really took off. The local fire engine went past with crew ringing the bell and flashing their blue light, and doing the same on their return. The man who collected the rubbish drove past on his way home and slowed down to shout that he was going home to fetch his wife. It was really good fun and when there was a sharp shower, who would have thought so many adults would have enjoyed jumping in puddles? The bar man was not the only one to be mortified. Millie chose to sit on a chair, staring out of the window at our antics, rather like a teenager unable to take in the shame of their parents' behaviour. This was a vital and joyous moment that Tony remembered and talked about for ever afterwards. Dementia is horrible and cruel, but life goes on and it is important, for all sorts of reasons, to grab and hold on to times like this and remember it is still possible to be wantonly happy.

6.

Being a carer

L ooking back now with the advantage of twenty-twenty hindsight, I can see how blissful ignorance can be, because it never really crossed my mind that I should not, or could not, be Tony's carer. I assumed it would be fairly straightforward; after all, Tony and I had known each other for a long time and, to be honest, sometimes his behaviour was so awful it didn't occur to me that Alzheimer's could make it any worse. In the early days of his illness my patience wasn't particularly tested, which allowed me to become perhaps a little too confident about my own caring abilities. By the time I was under real pressure I felt too emotionally committed to the situation to back out. As usual, when I find myself in a bit of a fix, it is my sheer bloody-mindedness that won't allow me to give in – I always want to see things through and sort it out. That, and the inescapable fact that despite the sometimes horrendous difficulties I faced, I loved the bones of the man and promised several times when he was frightened about what was happening to him that I wouldn't leave him.

My lack of awareness, combined with the absence of any real or particularly useful source of advice and information about future possibilities and choices when Tony was first diagnosed, added to the blind faith I had in my capabilities and fortitude. But then, even knowing what I know now, would I really have made different choices? Probably not.

Right from the start, it was always my intention to maintain our daily lives and routines. Dementia is an illness that affects the lives of an increasing number of people and their families and friends, and therefore urgently needs to be normalised. Cancer is shattering, heart disease is frightening, but as a society and as individuals we have learned to confront them. Can we now do the same with dementia, please? Normalising it would help reduce the fear around it and allow us to approach it like any other disease – as something that might happen to any one of us.

As a child, I remember being scared of the unkempt, smelly old lady who wandered down the road pulling her wheeled shopper and muttering to herself. My friends and I were convinced she was a witch, as she was clearly crazy. Sometimes, barbarous children that we were, rather than run away we would stand and torment her and even throw stones. I'm not certain the way we treat the elderly in our society currently is that far removed in cruelty from such horrible childhood behaviour. A controversial statement it may be, but television documentaries have exposed the worst of care homes and their indifferent, malignant behaviour. Indeed, as the 'care industry' booms, it feeds into our innate need to hide away from that which frightens us, or those whose problems we fail or don't want to understand. Inevitably, it's a case of 'out of sight, out of mind'. The way dementia is perceived and reacted to must change.

Tony and I were at each other's side as partners in the early days of his diagnosis, pausing only to make sure, as his illness progressed, whatever we were doing was not too tiring or demanding. So when in 2015 I was elected Mayor of Todmorden, there was no question about whether Tony would be my official Consort, despite some of my council colleagues thinking it might not be appropriate for someone with dementia to take on such a role. I could see no good reason why he shouldn't and I couldn't bear the thought of how hurt he would have been if I had chosen someone else. My only proviso was that if he was having the sort of day where he was being downright offensive or difficult, I wouldn't take him with me. Fortunately, that didn't happen too often as he loved dressing up and meeting people. When he was tired from an event I would fret I had made the wrong decision, but then what was the right decision? Should I have left him snoozing in an armchair for most of the day, physically stress-free but under-stimulated mentally; or did I do the right thing in getting him out and about, meeting people, doing things, whilst knowing ultimately it put more strain on his already frail heart? Was it to be either quantity or quality of life? It was not just Tony who would have to live with the consequences of those choices, but me too. I found being a carer involved a fair level of guilt about decisions made or not made, as the case may be. In the end, we are human beings who can only do our best – a truism which didn't help much at the time, but which I can see now is right.

It had been a surprise to be elected Mayor as I was adamant I didn't want to stand for council, and had only relented when told I had no chance of winning, given the unpopularity of Tony's daughter and her husband, by this stage the former Prime Minister. Indeed, the week of the election, I was away in the Scottish Borders while Tony was in respite care. I had taken myself off to Scotland along with the dogs, but how I managed to drive there from West Yorkshire I do not know. I was beside myself with tiredness.

I arrived at the cottage I'd rented in the early evening and instead of sensibly leaving unpacking the car to the following morning, I decided it had to be done immediately. It was only after closing the cottage door on the world that I started to cry. I do not cry very often, but this was unlike anything I had ever experienced before. It was as if my body were being ripped apart by the sheer force of my sobs. The noise I was making was horrible, unrecognisable. It was the sound of loss, pain, anger, grief, frustration and loneliness, as months of exhaustion and emotion came roaring out of me. Emotion I had kept under tight rein at home so as not to frighten or upset Tony and which, for my own sake, I could not usually give in to. By the time I was able to bring myself back under control, I was on the floor, my nose bleeding, my throat sore and my chest aching with the effort of breathing. My poor dogs were trying to nuzzle and comfort me, licking the wreckage of my face, but all I could do at that moment was to crawl into bed.

The next day the wind was up and the rain was lashing down, and I decided to go to the coast. I love the beach in rough weather, the raw power and exhilaration of the breakers lifting me out of myself and soothing my soul. It was the perfect antidote to the wild sorrows of the previous night. I was then in the right state of mind to spend the week pottering about, going for long walks with the dogs and in the evening sitting and reading in front of the log burner, a glass of red wine in hand. Red wine was and continues to be therapeutic. That and embracing healing peace and solitude.

This break had taught me a tough lesson. I had to learn to accept how much respite care for Tony was necessary for us both, and whilst other people could not be me, they were still capable of looking after him. I had hit rock bottom physically and mentally through exhaustion, foolishly not doing something about it much sooner, as my ever-present fear that something would happen to Tony whilst I wasn't there had prevented me. I was fortunate to find a local care home, Stansfield Hall, where I could leave Tony without any profound sense of guilt as he didn't mind staying there too much. The staff at the home were lovely and crucially there was very little staff turnover, helping to create a feeling of permanence and security.

It was a good twenty-four hours after collecting Tony and returning home before I knew I had been elected to the town council. I was so sure I couldn't win, I hadn't bothered to check the results. Not only was I elected, but I had the highest vote of anyone on the council. So much for having no chance. But now I could tell Tony he would be filling the Duke of Edinburgh role during my year as Mayor – hopefully without too many of the gaffes, although this was by no means certain. He was somewhat disappointed when he saw the Consort's 'chain', a ribbon with an ordinary-looking medal on the end, was not nearly as big and blingy as the Mayor's. There was a little bit of gold-and-jewels envy going on. Even when people could see I was the one in the mayoral chain, many times the instant assumption was that I was the Lady Mayoress and Tony was the Mayor. He enjoyed correcting them, saying, 'Oh no. I'm here to support my lady wife. I am the Mayoress.' He also had to wear his suit a great many more times than he had ever worn one in his life, repeatedly joking that Scousers only ever wore a suit when they were the accused.

Catherine Emberson, the Town Clerk, and her trusty lieutenant Sue Berry, the Assistant Town Clerk, were crucial to my ability and success in fulfilling the role of Mayor. I relied on them a great deal. At the time, Catherine was looking after her mother, who was frail and elderly, and our shared experience brought us together as friends as well as colleagues. At the beginning of my mayoral year, Catherine was making vague rumblings about retiring, but fortunately for me she decided to work for another year. The door to her office was always open, so members of the public as well as councillors could pop in and out for advice and support on any number of issues.

When I arrived for mayoral briefings, the first thing she did was put the kettle on before we had a brief chat and catch up. Then we would get down to business. The moral and emotional support she gave me during those first few minutes of every meeting reinforced my confidence in her and the knowledge she was there, backing me all the way. On Remembrance Sunday, knowing Tony would not have the strength to walk through town, she made sure he was at the war memorial when the procession arrived. It is the role of the mayoral Consort to lay the town council wreath and Catherine held Tony's elbow as he fulfilled his duty. Catherine and Sue went above and beyond to look after Tony and me.

One of the traditional duties of the Mayor in Todmorden is to attend the annual Rotary Club Charter, a black-tie event. Tony's one suit was a lounge suit, so not quite appropriate. Chatting to Catherine about it, I suggested hiring a dinner suit for him. She was horrified, insisting it was out of the question; he simply had to have a new suit. It takes about thirty minutes on the train to get from Todmorden to Manchester; however,

Tony was no longer fit enough to walk from the station to the shops, so his disabled parking badge was a blessing. I could park the car as close as possible to the required shop, in this case Marks & Spencer, and prepare myself for a fraught experience. Any brownie points I might have accumulated in heaven were about to be lost.

The first issue to be addressed was Tony's unwillingness to own a suit, let alone wear one. I was eventually able to get him to understand how important it was to his role as my Consort. I had chosen M&S as their assistants are usually helpful, if, at times, a little difficult to locate. I explained what we wanted and Tony was taken to the fitting rooms to be measured. I tagged along behind, much to the consternation of other chaps trying on clothes. Their wives were waiting dutifully outside, but no matter how helpful the assistant, he was unlikely to be used to dealing with someone with dementia.

I also needed to make sure Tony behaved. Despite my insistence that he had to have a suit, once out of my sight, Tony would almost certainly try to persuade the assistant otherwise. By this point, I had learned to be very straight about Tony's illness and simply explained to the assistant that my husband had dementia and my assistance was necessary. Nevertheless, it was the usual nightmare, with the poor assistant caught in the middle of me being assertive and not allowing any nonsense from Tony, and Tony telling him what a bully I was and how he needed protecting from me. Eventually, the shop assistant and I had Tony smartly kitted out. For all the physical devastation that dementia and heart disease were causing, he was still a handsome man. I had appealed to the theatrical side of Tony's personality by finding a dress shirt with a wing collar and tiny pleats down the front. He looked fantastic. By the time I had paid for everything, we were both in desperate need of tea and cake – our perennial reward for surviving a difficult task. I suspect the unfortunate assistant was looking for something a little stronger.

And thus we arrived at the Rotary Club Charter dinner with me in a little black number and Tony in a dinner suit. No one could have suspected the trauma we'd gone through to get to this point, but that was a thing of the past. Now I had to ensure our evening would pass without any incidents; and if that was not possible, then please make them only little ones! It was Tony's loss of social inhibition rather than his repetitive telling of stories that could startle the unprepared. Not that he had much inhibition in the first place. Someone who was prepared to get their kit off on a nightly basis in front of a theatre audience was unlikely to be hampered by shyness. When he was chatting to people, I would worry about the appropriateness of some of his stories if I was not on hand to intervene and rapidly change the subject. But usually Tony's stories were welcome and provoked raucous laughter from the predominantly male group gathered around him. He was born to perform and his dementia didn't take that away from him.

On this occasion, we were seated at the top table for dinner and things seemed to be going smoothly, until Tony started to get bored and sleepy. The room was very warm and we had eaten a rather large meal. Tony wanted to go home and he wanted me to go with him. He began a campaign of persistently elbowing me in the ribs, gently at first, but then not so gently. When that tactic failed, he upped the ante by taking his watch off, laying on the table in front of me and starting to tap it after first nudging me with his elbow.

Drastic action was needed. I picked up the watch and he looked at me to see what I was going to do. I gave him the full-on look, the look women in general but mothers in particular perfect which stops miscreants in their tracks. Other diners must have seen what was happening, but I had learned simply to take control of a situation without betraying my embarrassment. After all, I am the oldest of five and the mother of four sons, and assertiveness is in my DNA, so there was no way I was ever going to take the meek and mild route. I have been called a witch, a harridan, a bossy bitch and much worse labels reserved for women, by those who have no understanding of what it takes to look after and support someone living with dementia, or those who just hate strong women. Nevertheless, Tony sensibly retreated and, with only a few minutes more of speeches, we ended the evening on a high note and could mark it down as a success.

*

If only other aspects of our life with dementia had proved that straightforward. Caring for a loved one with Alzheimer's is hard enough. On top of that, our finances were a nightmare – mostly because it would appear to be the policy of government departments and local councils not to give out details of what you are entitled to in a situation like ours. If you don't know, you don't get, because no one is going to volunteer any information beyond what you've asked for. It's a bit like the answers I gave my sons when they were little and asked about sex without knowing that was what they were talking about. As I didn't want to overwhelm them with science, I simply answered the question they asked. It was when they were older I gave them the really vital advice about choices and always making sure it was covered in rubber. The difference in our situations was I was a parent guiding my children. The Department for Work and Pensions (DWP), however, seemed to be denying knowledge to adults who desperately needed it.

Answering the same set of questions for different administrative assistants in different departments, as you are passed from pillar to post, is time-consuming and soul destroying. But even that level of recognition depends on discovering who you need to be talking to in the first place, and exactly which bit of the process they are knowledgeable about. Having broken into the system to the point where I could have a telephone assessment of Tony's eligibility for further benefits on top of his state pension, I was faced with another level of complexity. I explained that Tony still occasionally received royalties or residuals from films and television repeats, but this income depended entirely on the whim of television schedulers. After some discussion, when it became clear this really wasn't any form of regular income, they decided we would rightly be entitled to extra financial support.

That worked well until some time later, when I received a further call from the DWP. Tony had had a reasonably good year in terms of payments and this had come to the notice of the DWP, who were now concerned there might be fraud going on. Obviously, this was all fair enough, but did the tone of their questioning have to be quite so belligerent? Once I realised the purpose of the call, I attempted to explain to the person at the other end of the line that their colleague had decided to discount what were intermittent and usually small payments. I was told I was not telling the truth as I would never have been given such advice.

Ignoring everything I was trying to say, the woman then insisted on speaking to Tony to make certain he agreed to me representing him. I explained he had Alzheimer's and would have no idea what she was talking about. She continued to insist and I continued to refuse until she actually looked at her notes and saw I had power of attorney, giving me legal authorisation to act on his behalf. Having resolved that matter, the conversation went round and round until she was convinced the residual payments were not a regular source of income. We finally agreed that Tony would continue to receive the benefits he had been given and was entitled to.

Yet no apology was forthcoming for her initially aggressive attitude or the nasty assumption that I was trying to defraud the benefit system. I consider myself to be reasonably intelligent and articulate but that was a difficult and unpleasant situation to deal with, so goodness knows how people without the benefit of my education and life experience cope. I wanted to shout with frustration, so I understand perfectly how people are driven to aggression and even violence by a system that appears to be deliberately and cruelly punitive. It was my choice to look after Tony, but I certainly didn't expect to be punished for it or to face unpleasant accusations. A little respect rather than suspicion would have been welcome. I now understand Kafka's novel *The Castle* and its overwhelming sense of dislocation, as the protagonist battles with unhelpful authorities, far better than I was ever able to when studying it at school.

My resolve and tenacity to be Tony's carer were tested to breaking point when I realised that, rather than recognising a carer's huge contribution to health and social wellbeing, government policy often appears to be predicated on the perverse notion that as individuals we are a drain on welfare budgets. So, you might imagine my astonishment when I discovered the National Dementia Strategy in England, published as long ago as 2009, has a goal of supporting people with dementia in their own homes as it costs less than having them live in a care home. Would anyone mind if I just scream now?

More recent research into this particular aspect of looking after those with dementia has made the same point. A Finnish study, published in 2013, revealed that elderly people living in a care home cost the state €25,300 each annually; a combination of formal and informal care costs €22,300; whilst a person living at home cared for by a family member, i.e. an informal caregiver, costs the state €4,900. Although it's true that the figures for formal care have sky-rocketed in recent years to an average of £30,000 per person in the UK, jumping to £40,000 if any nursing is required, the fundamental point remains the same. As these costs continue to escalate, informal caregivers save the state an awful lot of money, as even without any formal healthcare education of their own, they are caring for, or helping, a person with functional disabilities, prolonged psychiatric or physical illness, or age-related problems. In other words, an awful lot of bang for your buck.

But these sorts of figures look only at public costs. The hidden cost is when you are faced, as I was, with the collapse of a household income as it becomes based on benefits. The care I gave willingly to Tony was 24/7, but I was not entitled to any benefits in my own name, let alone perceived as worthy of even a minimum wage. I haven't yet been able to find a website with research showing the average yearly loss of earned income for a carer. It seems that, for all the government reviews and promises, this issue has yet to become a serious consideration. Although it won't make any difference to me now, I still find it almost unbearable to think that carers will in all likelihood carry on struggling with this most basic issue for years to come, even as the care-home system buckles and collapses under the strain that our ageing population will inevitably place on it.

A fair income for carers would help ease their financial stress and recognise that, in the current situation, it is little wonder people who try to care for a loved one at home often simply give up when it is this hard. Living in a house where every penny counts does not help to create the calm and positive atmosphere essential for everyone's wellbeing, especially those living with dementia.

What the care system doesn't need are any more quick fixes dressed up as real change and languishing on some government minister's to-do list. What it does need is compassionate, innovative and forward-thinking policy-making that encompasses grassroots as well as top-down solutions. There is far too much of our being told what is good for us either by the government or by any of the organisations who claim to be on our side. It is now well overdue for carers to have an opportunity to make their contribution to healthcare policy, express their opinions based on real-life experience, and be heard rather than politely listened to and then forgotten about.

Dementia care, like the rest of the National Health Service, needs to have politics removed from its policy making. With an increasingly ageing population and a shrinking work force, dementia is a critical issue facing the government; it's an economic and health time bomb that successive administrations have chosen to ignore. As a society, we are now reaping the fallout of that particular failure. I believe the creation of a cross-party panel, with the specific purpose of devising sustainable, far-reaching and workable dementia policy, is now the only way forward. This cross-party panel must also include a proportionate number of carers and people with dementia as well as health and research professionals. Government and the NHS might have the money and the drugs, but carers have the experience.

It is foolish to go on dismissing the knowledge and experience of carers as simply anecdotal. The government policy of austerity has seen local councils chop back their social service budgets to the bone – in many cases to the legal limit. As usual, it is the most vulnerable who have paid the price.

I know what a lifeline day centres can be in providing regular weekly respite, but these centres are now in danger of having to limit places further, if not actually closing down. This makes no economic or social sense when families under pressure decide they can no longer cope and are pushed into deciding that the person they are caring for has to go into a home. If a place is available, that is. There is an obscene amount of pressure on families and individuals, often hidden from view, as the government and dementia organisations focus on the holy grail of research. 'Jam tomorrow' never was and never will be a good enough slogan.

At the point of diagnosis, dementia carers need clear and easily accessible information, which provides details of everything we might need to know, and thereby removes the anxious and at times overwhelming need to search for knowledge and support. Such resources may be in production somewhere, but I've not come across one yet – and they need to be provided by the DWP and widely available in all the places carers might go, such as doctors' surgeries, dentists, day centres, libraries, social services departments, solicitors' offices and schools. In the end, my reality – and I'm sure it is true for many other dementia carers – was that coping with Tony was often easier than coping with the DWP, local council services, the medical profession, social services, well-meaning but uninformed bystanders and anyone else who might have an opinion about what was best for us.

As time went on, I found myself between a rock and a hard place, coping with the equally draining demands of an unheeding officialdom and Tony's increasing confusion over the simplest tasks, such as getting showered and dressed, or getting undressed for bed.

'Do I need to take everything off?'

'Yes.'

'What, everything?'

'Yes. Everything.'

'Then what do I do?'

'Just get your kit off and we'll take it from there.'

'Should I leave my socks on?'

'Why? Are you cold?'

'No.'

'Take them off then.'

This process would take ages and involve several encouraging prompts when he forgot if he was getting dressed or undressed. The desire to just do it for him, so it was sorted quickly, had to be firmly resisted, but – as mentioned – I'm not famed for my patience. Getting dressed into his pyjamas became easier for Tony when I swapped the pyjama jacket for an old T-shirt. Buttons were tough as he had big hands, his fine motor control was diminishing, and also fastening the buttons in the right holes was too difficult.

In the last few months before Tony died, he became anxious about having a shower. Every morning, I would protect the bathroom floor with old towels as we had to keep the shower door open so I could see what was happening and he could see me and feel safer. We tried all sorts of equipment like shower seating, but then the problem was getting him back on to his feet, because, even with a safety mat, we would both be sliding around. I think perhaps it was the water that worried him, as I would insist he got himself under the shower head. He would then start roaring and I would be telling him to be quiet and to put his hand out while I squirted some shower gel into it, so he could wash his hair. He would then promptly soap up his tummy or anywhere but where I'd asked, while I stood there soaked to the bone, trying to get some soap on to his head and encouraging him to wash his face. This daily drama would only last a few minutes, but it could well have been a lifetime given the stress of flooding, soap and sometimes choice of language.

If showering was tough, nothing could beat shaving for trauma. Oh my, the way he carried on and tried to provoke me, I'm surprised he let me anywhere near his throat with a razor in my hand. If I shaved up, he wanted me to shave down. If I shaved down, he wanted me to shave up. Eventually, I ignored all of his 'suggestions' and just got on with the job in hand – until I decided it was going to be far easier for him to grow a beard, a strategy he was happy with and had been advocating for some time. This worked well until, bored with the itchiness of facial hair, he had a go at shaving himself. His face was covered in cuts and the wash basin was a blood bath. It was allegedly all my fault for not shaving him anymore – and did he have to do everything himself? Just look at what I had made him do.

Help was at hand when Phil, the barber in Todmorden market, agreed to give Tony a hot towel shave whenever he had his hair cut. I would leave Tony with him and get a cup of coffee whilst he sorted Tony out. The everyday thoughtfulness from the people around us helped to make our lives run that little bit more smoothly and offered me temporary relief.

Tony liked going out. In fact, right up to the time when he took to his bed, only a couple of weeks before he died, we would head out together once or sometimes twice a week. As well as visiting gardens, Tony enjoyed going for drives in the car, which gave him the opportunity to see things he wouldn't otherwise get to see, like lambing time on the hills around our home – big softy that he was.

There was, however, a terrifying moment on the motorway. We were sitting in a traffic jam on the M6 when Tony suddenly decided to get out of the car. I didn't spot immediately what he was doing, though fortunately the driver in the car next to us did.

'What the hell do you think you were doing, you complete screaming idiot?' were my first words to Tony when he was safely back in the vehicle.

'I was bored,' he replied.

I lashed back, 'You've got dementia – you can't get bored!'

Sympathy was not my first reaction when he had just frightened me half to death. Looking after someone with dementia can demand thinking of every possible eventuality, but for heaven's sake, how could I have anticipated him doing that?

*

In order to be able to carry on doing things with Tony, I was constantly rejigging our finances, sometimes postponing paying bills in order to go somewhere with him. I figured that could always be dealt with later. Then Lydia, Tony's social worker, told me about and subsequently arranged direct payments for us. Life and finances became much easier. The arrangement was assessed each year and the payments were paid directly into a bank account for Tony's care provision. The money was paid by the council's social services department with the aim of giving me more flexibility over how Tony's care and support were arranged and provided. I interpreted this to mean it was money to help me look after him, caring for him in the way I felt was the most suitable and supportive. I used the money for respite care; to take him on holiday; to make the garden more accessible for him; for days out and to go out for lunch. I also used the money to keep the car running, or how else would I have been able to do any of these things?

I occasionally even used the direct payment fund to pay the mortgage when an unexpected bill came up and money was just too tight. Keeping a roof over our heads was, I believed, a vital part of caring for him. If I couldn't do that, he would have to go into a home despite what either of us wanted or my efforts to keep him living with me. However, it would appear that Calderdale Council's definition of care and mine were not terribly similar. The Council's definition seemed to turn on a very narrow and prescriptive idea, whilst mine was much more flexible and focused on Tony's specific needs. I assumed that if they were happy for me to be saving them thousands of pounds a year by looking after Tony at home, they would also be happy to assume that I was sensible enough to spend the direct payments on providing quality of life for Tony. I didn't get that one quite right, but at least they waited for Tony to die before challenging my spending decisions. They were marginally more thoughtful than the council tax official who, when I spoke to her a few weeks after Tony's death, told me they should really have been informed of Tony's death on the day he died.

One of the holidays that I took Tony on was with our friends Maggie and Matthew, who live in Liverpool; Maggie was always known to Tony as 'Liverpool Maggie'. I first met her at the University of Salford where she was the Pro Vice Chancellor for External Affairs and also, more importantly for me, Dean of the College for Health and Social Care. Her role in helping the university to set up the Salford Institute for Dementia was fundamental to its initial success. We became good friends as she encouraged me to take my experiences with Tony and turn them into something powerful and positive by speaking, lecturing and writing about them – shining a light on the too often forgotten lived reality of people with dementia and their carers.

I was once asked to speak to a group of consultant psychologists who were, of course, absolutely up to speed on the latest scientific and medical developments in dementia research. I, on the other hand, was fully up to speed on living with and caring full-time for someone with Alzheimer's. We inhabited parallel universes and it was interesting to discuss with them how those universes might be bridged. I don't think anything ever came out of our discussions, which is a great shame as there was perhaps the possibility of creating a shared forward momentum on developing holistic dementia strategies. I sometimes worry that the story of dementia is doomed to be the story of such lost opportunities.

On this occasion, we rented a cottage with Maggie, Matthew and their daughter Tessa in the Scottish Borders on the banks of the River Tweed. It was an idyllic spot, beautiful and isolated, and the weather was also kind to us given it was October. A few days earlier Tony had celebrated his eighty-fourth birthday with a surprise party I arranged for him. He was still on a bit of a high, although I don't think he remembered why, but it was one of the good times. There were some lovely walks around the cottage and although these were out of the question for Tony, he could sit in the garden with Matthew, who also smoked. Maggie, Matthew and Tessa were endlessly patient and kind with Tony. I can't repeat often enough how vital the support of all our good friends was and how much I remain grateful for their friendship and love.

Maggie and I are both quilters and we took Tony with us as we explored the Borders Quilt Trail. We had a great time fuelling our obsessional tendencies as we oohed and aahed over, fondled and bought even more fabric to add to our collections. Meanwhile, Tony was very happy to be fussed over by the shop assistants, who gave him cups of tea and occasionally, if he was particularly lucky, slices of cake. It was a perfect arrangement.

There's no point pretending that looking after Tony wasn't often hard, lonely and frustrating, but because he was living at home, we were able to share the happy times and moments that would have otherwise been lost to us – such as going on holiday together, like we did in the Scottish Borders. As time has gone on and Tony's death feels a little less emotionally raw, it is those memories that now make me smile and hug myself; sometimes through tears, but the memories are always there as a comfort.

Affection is always important in any close relationship and as Tony's physical health and mental capacity declined it became even more important for us. Hugs and kisses were an essential part of our communication with each other, showing that love remained between us and we were literally still in touch. A continued sexual relationship, however, was much more problematic. There seems to be a general assumption that older people don't indulge in such activities anyway, but when one person has dementia there is the added complication of consent and how to know it has been freely given.

I am aware there has been a lot of academic and welfare research into the issue of consent and rights in care homes where couples are still living together, or when people meet in a care home and then become a couple. In that situation, there are professionals within the home who can provide appropriate help and advice and make sure any sexual relationship is consensual. Where a couple are living in their own home, the questions are different and it is down to the non-dementia person to make what can be difficult moral choices about consent.

When Tony was first diagnosed, this was not one of our problems; but it gradually became one and I tied myself into philosophical and emotional knots, attempting to work out and balance our needs and choices. Consent is fundamental to any loving relationship and given the horrors I went through with my father's violent and incestuous behaviour, it was something that bothered me greatly. In the end, it involved another one of our 'muddle through' resolutions. Tony's heart problems made him too tired for any kind of physical exertion and I think sex was one of those things, like smoking, he gradually forgot he did and enjoyed. This was pretty much fine for me, although what I did miss was not so much the sex itself as the intimacy of being together, enclosed entirely in our own private world. It was one more thing we lost to dementia and another reason why I rail against the idea that one can 'live well' with dementia. This, I believe, is an advertising gimmick designed to make us feel better about dementia, while masking the reality of the lack of progress on finding the causes and dealing with outcomes. 'Living well' may be possible in the early days, or for those whose dementia doesn't really progress from their initial diagnosis, but for those of us who travel further, there is real suffering. How can it not be when so much is lost?

7.

Life as we knew it

My son Matthew lives in France, where he married his partner, Capucine, or Capu as she is known by family and friends, in August 2014. Capu was born and brought up in Brittany, so that is where the wedding was to be held. There was going to be a civil ceremony in Pénestin, followed by lunch in an excellent restaurant, before heading back to her family home for a garden party in the evening.

Matthew asked me to make bunting for the garden and as I have the magpie acquisitiveness of all quilters, I initially didn't think that would be a problem. That is, until they told me they needed forty-six metres of it. Surely even my kleptomaniac tendencies with fabric couldn't extend that far? It seems they did, though, as I dragged out various bits and pieces I'd been saving for years, waiting for the right moment. ... It took three days to cut out all the triangles, as rather than use a rotary cutter and board, I used pinking shears to stop the cotton fraying. Tony was tasked with putting the triangles into piles according to fabric. He was surprisingly patient and didn't get bored as he was pleased I had found a way for him to help. He also had a moment when his brain sparked with an original idea and he suggested that as well as sorting the triangles into relevant piles, he should pin them into groups of ten. It was good to be working together again on a project. It was almost like the pre-dementia days and I could pretend for a little while things were still fine.

Eventually, the bunting was completed and I turned my attention to organising our trip to France. Our friend Chris was travelling with us and we also had three dogs to pack into the car, along with our luggage and wedding finery. Although I later discovered French women don't tend to wear hats at weddings, I had indulged myself with a far too expensive hat from the lovely milliners in Hebden Bridge. It was in a large hat box and I probably made the journey much more difficult than it should have been by constantly reminding my fellow passengers to be aware of and not crush the box.

We stayed overnight near Thame before driving to Dover to catch the ferry to Calais. The dogs travelled together in the boot space, but when we arrived at Dover I decided to move Carol, our elderly rescue Cavalier King Charles Spaniel, on to the back seat where she would not be mithered by the other dogs during the crossing. When we returned to the car to disembark, I noticed straightaway that something was wrong with Carol. I got into the car and could see she was dead. Scrambling back out, I told Tony and Chris. Chris immediately burst into tears and Tony told me not to be so stupid. I looked at them both, wondering what to do, when Tony made the utterly brilliant suggestion we throw the dog overboard. Treating him to my best withering look, I suggested they both get in the car while I sorted out Carol. After wrapping her in a fleece blanket, I put her into the back of the car with the other two dogs and prayed they would be indifferent to the body now occupying part of their space. Once we were on the road out of the ferry port, I phoned Matthew and asked him to dig a grave for Carol. He was a little surprised, but agreed.

I was driving straight from Calais to Brittany, a journey of some time and distance, but a diet of water, chewing gum and music were the key to keeping me going. I knew things were going to be difficult as we had hardly got on the road before Tony, who was in the back, started tapping me on the shoulder to inform me there was a dead dog in the boot of the car. I told him I knew and he wasn't to worry about it, as I would sort it out soon, but his dementia made him obsess about the dog and also forget I had told him I would deal with it as soon as I could. This was going to be, in so many ways, a long journey.

Things only got worse when after a couple of hours we were treated to one of those spectacular thunder and lightning storms France specialises in during the summer months. The torrential rain meant I had to slow right down to a crawl when I had hoped to complete this journey as soon as humanly possible. Chris tried to cheer me up by telling me that at least the lightning couldn't electrocute us as the car was a Faraday cage. This information was of no comfort to me as at that point electrocution looked like the soft option. The tapping on my shoulder increased exponentially as Tony demanded to know why I had slowed down, because we were never going to get there at this rate – and did I know there was a dead dog in the back of the car?

I finished the journey with almost a full packet of Wrigley's Spearmint stuffed into my mouth: as I was chomping on the gum with such ferocity, Chris became worried I might break my teeth, so she kept feeding me more and more pieces to lessen the impact on my molars. It was just before midnight when I drove up the driveway. Capu's dad, Jean Hubert, was standing in a pool of light from the house with a gin and tonic in his hand, which he gave me almost before I turned off the engine. In that moment I fell in love with the man.

The first thing Tony said to Jean Hubert was, 'Do you know there's a dead dog in the back of our car?'

Matthew had dug a grave for Carol and we buried her wrapped in her blanket. Poor old girl, she would have loved the adventure and the beach was just five minutes' walk away.

There was plenty to do in the days before the wedding. On the basis I had once done evening classes in flower arranging, I was charged with putting together the wedding flowers – everything from table decorations to Capu's bouquet. Thank goodness the theme was English village wedding as it would hide a multitude of mistakes and not-quite-rights.

Capu and I spent a pleasant morning in a flower whole-saler's, choosing flowers. Gypsophilia was her main choice, along with roses, freesias and lavender. Tony, meanwhile, was back at the house indulging in a favourite pastime: sitting in the garden, basking in sunshine. He hadn't wanted to come with Capu and me, which was fair enough. He liked flowers, but not enough to put up with women trailing around making decisions. I didn't realise at the time that it was an indicator of how tired he was, not just the tiredness that needs sleep, but the tiredness that comes with illness and his heart deteriorating.

Something else I had to take on board was that his focus had moved on from the dead dog in the back of the car to: 'Where is Carol?' Each time he asked, which was often, and was told she had died, he would become upset as every time it was a revelation. I decided it might perhaps be a good idea to mark her grave with a bush of some sort, so a hydrangea was bought and Tony was involved in its planting. I was hopeful this might help and to some extent it did. When he asked where the dog was, we could point to the spot in the garden and say, 'Come on, you know where she is, you helped to plant the bush.' He would nod and agree, though I don't know how much he remembered, but being reminded was helpful – not quite the same as telling him she was dead.

I started putting the flowers together two days before the wedding. I had no idea it would be such hard work, but I loved doing it. People wandered in and out of the garage where I was working to bring drinks, chat and look at what

I was doing. Everyone except Tony, who claimed the garage was too cold to visit even for a moment. He could be such a wuss!

I finished the flowers and as there was a festival in a nearby town that evening, it was decided we should all relax by going there to have something to eat. By this time, the day before the wedding, our friends Brian and Betty had arrived. The English contingent – Brian, Betty, Chris, Tony and me – all set off in the same car supposedly in convoy with everyone else, but we soon became separated. We managed to find a parking space, but as the town was busy it was quite some way out from the centre.

Our little group set off, but we made fairly slow progress as Chris uses a stick and Tony was no longer able to walk at any great pace. I was soon getting text messages from Matthew, urging us to hurry up as they were waiting. I realised he would be a little nervous the night before his wedding, so I just let him know we would be there as soon as possible. The texts kept coming in ever greater numbers, but I was caught in an impossible situation. Brian and Betty were increasingly concerned about Tony and felt the walk was too much for him and we should turn back.

Eventually, I went on ahead to find my son and everyone else to explain the problems we were having. Matthew was angry and upset things weren't going to plan as I had to tell him the rest of us could not make it to the harbour and that we were going back to Pénestin for something to eat. I was beyond tired trying to cope with everything, torn between the needs of Tony and Matthew.

The day of the wedding, Betty and Brian (after a lifetime of working as teachers) were organised and ready to go over to Jean Hubert's well before the rest of us, so they went off. We were going to be delayed as Tony was refusing to get out of bed. I knew he was really tired from the previous night, but still hoped to persuade him. Nothing would move him and all my frustration from the previous night became displaced on to him as I yelled about how selfish, stupid and thoughtless he was being. How could he do this to me when I had driven all this way and worked so hard, helping with wedding preparations? He simply rolled over and told me to fuck off – behaviour I had become familiar with as his dementia worsened. Chris, who has always been a rock, suggested I get ready and go to my son's wedding and leave Tony where he wanted to be. So that's what I did.

Betty told me later that when she arrived at the house, Matthew was concerned I might still be upset about his reaction the night before and might even decide not to come to the wedding. When I arrived he greeted me with a big hug and, of course, there had never been any question of me not attending.

After the beautiful wedding at the town hall in Pénestin, I went back to the house, where Tony was in a much better mood and tempted by the prospect of a good meal. He showered and dressed and we set off together for the wedding lunch. He was wearing the buttonhole I had made him and he was up for a party. People were pleased to see him when he arrived and within a short while he had forgotten all about his earlier refusal to accompany me. The rest of our stay in Brittany went off with minimal fuss, but to be honest I was quite relieved to go home. Familiar surroundings for Tony made my life much easier.

Once back home, the plan had been for Tony to resume his routine of day centre visits, but after his first day back, he looked completely ashen and was clearly not well. I called an ambulance and on the advice of the paramedics, he was taken off to hospital. Tony was admitted for observation and I believed from what I was told by the medical staff that this was routine practice and he would be discharged the next day. When I called the hospital the following morning he had already been transferred to a medical ward. I visited him that afternoon and he seemed fine and keen to go home. The doctor I spoke to said nothing to dispel this notion, telling me Tony had been moved on to this ward as the bed in the first ward was needed.

The next day, Tony started to deteriorate and more serious investigations were needed. After a few more days, I was called into the consultant's office for an end-of-life conversation. Tests had revealed Tony had chronic heart failure and other symptoms of COPD (chronic obstructive pulmonary disease) and the doctor was not certain whether Tony would survive beyond the next twenty-four hours. Did we have any plans in place? We did, but the rapidness from which we had gone from Tony's possibly coming home tomorrow to having this conversation left me gasping and shaken. I wanted to be calm and collected, if only to prove I could be an adult about it, but I was struggling.

No matter how many times you discuss someone's wishes, it is still no preparation for the reality of being asked these sorts of question. I would, of course, honour Tony's requests for a peaceful departure, but there was still a tiny, insistent voice in my head telling me I didn't have to. Who would know if I said or did anything necessary to keep him alive? The answer was, I would know and I would have to live the rest of my life knowing I had failed him at this most crucial time.

I told the doctor that Tony wanted no bells and whistles, no bright lights nor panoply of medical interventions, but a simple, calm ending. We agreed that, if there was the time and opportunity, Tony would be brought home to die and, if not, I would be given the maximum time possible to reach the hospital. Like so many others facing this situation, I didn't want him to die alone.

At home that night, I made lots of promises to God – if only He would let Tony recover and come home. I promised to be nice to everyone, even those I didn't like; I would never again forget to buy cat treats and inflict dog biscuits on the cats instead; really, whatever He wanted as long as we could square this deal. I think I must have put myself into hock with Him for at least the next century, but my prayers were answered and Tony did come home. His life force was extraordinary, but he never regained his spark; he was much quieter and more passive and that made me sad. I think this was probably the point I realised I had lost my husband and my mourning began.

Yet I was not prepared to let him sit quietly in a chair and die, disengaged from the world. We would still be companions and a physical presence in each other's lives. I managed to get Tony out and about regularly, either to the day centre or by taking him out for a few hours myself. Although he didn't eat much, he enjoyed going out for lunch because it was as much the familiarity and the routine as the food that pleased him. We had a circuit of places he liked where he was known and the staff were familiar with his menu preferences and were happy to chat with him. Tony's top choice was the Apricot Meringue in Clitheroe, where he was always greeted with much fuss and pleasure by his favourite waitresses, Caroline and Linda, who would also ask me how I was doing and hug me when we were leaving. I appreciated their thoughtfulness as I was usually – as carers often are – the invisible one. We would then have a short amble around Clitheroe, usually taking in the sweetie shop where Tony would indulge his chocolate habit and I would buy gummy bears.

As I mentioned, I first began to notice Tony's early signs of confusion when he mixed fact with fiction in the novels he read, but by now we had moved on considerably from that point. Back then, he could still enjoy a book, but now we were at a stage where he could no longer read as he couldn't remember the last sentence, let alone the last paragraph or chapter. Yet we still went to bookshops as they were one of his favourite places and he still chose books for himself, which I knew would never be read; but the main thing was that he was out and connecting socially and making choices to a certain extent. He was holding on to words, still valuing their importance to him; how many thousands had he spoken and remembered through his life and career? Reading to him was the answer, mainly short poems he recalled from his childhood and later life. I would also read Shakespeare to him, which he could still quote extensively – he always regretted not having had the opportunity to play King Lear. I think he would have made a fine Lear or perhaps a Prospero.

And we continued to go to the cinema together, something we had always enjoyed. We were regulars at the Hebden Bridge Picture House. Mostly, Tony fell asleep because it was warm and dark and he'd lost track of the plot. I was content as long as he didn't start to snore. Driving home, I would tell him the story, which was fine as the most important thing was that we had been out together, doing 'normal' things.

There was, though, one film we went to see that really grabbed Tony and during which he stayed awake and focused until the end. He was even talking about it the next morning, a by now unheard of feat of memory. Although it was a good film, I have no idea what it was about *Calvary* with Brendan Gleeson that so completely electrified Tony. He didn't stop talking about it even when we went to bed and I just had to hope he would run out of steam, so I could get some rest.

We had gone through a difficult patch during which Tony was very wakeful at night, so I'd moved into the other bedroom in the quest for sleep. All that happened then was that Tony came into the room and woke me up, mostly wanting to know why I wasn't in our bed. In desperation one night, I locked the door so he couldn't get in. The result was even worse as he stood outside the bedroom door crying, wanting to know why he couldn't reach me. I gave up on this strategy and tried to use the days Tony was at the day centre to catch up on sleep. Respite breaks were also a good survival technique. Tony was still not keen, but he no longer got himself into a total strop about it, particularly after I found Stansfield Hall for him, close to where we lived.

I didn't always go away when Tony was in respite care, often preferring to be at home and catch up with myself (and sleep). However, in July 2017, I decided to go to Israel as I have friends in Tel Aviv. It was the hottest time of the year in the Middle East, but I wanted to get away to a far-off land; and the sunshine and heat would be welcome after a dreary West Yorkshire winter. I did worry what I would do if Tony should die whilst I was away, but I also knew it was essential for my own wellbeing to have a complete break. These two needs were a constant source of tension in my life. Thinking about my decision now, I believe at some level I knew what was coming. Tony was really frail and his end could not be too far away; and I would need all my strength, physically and emotionally, to cope with what would be a tough and painful period of my life.

Israel is an interesting and beautiful country, although somewhat paranoid – inevitably, I suppose. I was based in Tel Aviv, but I spent two days in Jerusalem where I stayed in the American Colony Hotel. I was anticipating a real treat but was sadly disappointed, although when I first arrived I was delighted to see Mary Beard and her husband were also checking in. I'm afraid I behaved like some over-excited fan rather than the cool, sophisticated person I would like to be seen as. I still squirm when I think about it, but they were both lovely and friendly.

During my stay at the hotel, I went to have a cup of tea and refreshments in the pretty courtyard, but failed to attract the attention of a waiter, so I had to go over to where the waiters were standing about and chatting to order. No cutlery arrived with my panna cotta and when I wanted to leave I was once again roundly ignored, so I got up and went to my room. A little while later, the restaurant manager was knocking on my door to tell me I should not have left the courtyard without signing my room bill. I was angry and really upset to be treated in this way, particularly given the poor service I had received: the problem would not have arisen if the waiters had been doing their job properly.

When he had gone I had a furious debate with myself: should I feel humiliated and cry, or should I complain? A glass of water, a few deep breaths and down I went to see the hotel manager. He was somewhat surprised to hear what I had to say, but I managed to maintain a calm and dignified manner, ending my complaint with a flourish by telling him I would never recommend his hotel to anyone – particularly a woman travelling alone. Feeling rather satisfied with myself, I stepped back and almost fell on to a low table behind me. Gathering myself, I walked off, clutching my book, to the garden for an early supper of pizza and wine. As I sat down at a table, struggling to hold back tears, I realised just how much looking after Tony all this time had taken out of me. What had happened to my self-confidence? Why had I allowed myself to be treated in this rude and uncivil way? And why was I crying about it? Probably because I was exhausted and my self-belief had, like Elvis, left the building. I usually don't cry; I would far rather sort things out than cry about them.

Apart from when I got on the wrong bus to travel back to Tel Aviv, the rest of my stay was uneventful. My lovely friends Emanuela and Yona were very hospitable and I met a lot of interesting people. I must confess, though, a favourite memory is sitting on the beach in Tel Aviv at midnight, eating chips and drinking beer. I went home feeling rested, happier and braced for whatever was coming next. I would need to be.

*

When I picked Tony up from respite care, he had noticeably declined to a much greater extent than usual following a stay there. He was physically frailer and his confusion much more noticeable, although he did recognise me as soon as I walked in, which was a good sign. This was the last time Tony would go into respite care and it took me much longer to get him back into the routines of home. It was interesting how, as I eased him back into being at home, his sense of connection with people and his surroundings would also improve – probably because he was getting individual and focused care.

As usual, we spent a lot of time in the garden on the bench by our wildlife pond. It was a calm and soothing space for both of us, where he would tell me his stories for the zillionth time and I would ask questions as if I had never heard them before. Sitting there one afternoon, he suddenly asked me where all the frogs had gone. Startled out of my semi-doze, I said I didn't know, but they were probably in the pond somewhere.

'Where?'

'I don't know – in the water somewhere, or hiding by the rocks.'

'I don't believe you. I think you've killed them all.'

Being accused of having an affair was one thing, but massacring frogs was quite another: 'Don't be ridiculous,' I said.

'I'm sure it's illegal to kill frogs, I might have to talk to our Cherie about this,' was his response.

Bonkers though this conversation was, he was being completely serious and the only strategy was to divert him from thoughts of amphibian annihilation. 'Would you like me to go and make some tea?' I asked and immediately his thoughts were transferred to the possibility of chocolate biscuits with the tea.

I had learned to live with the surreal parallel universe that is dementia. The solution was not to challenge or question – there was no point – but to roll with whatever came from left-field.

In August our friend Ernst was over from Austria and he was going to stay with us for a few days. Tony didn't initially recognise Ernst and Ernst was shocked by Tony's appearance. He was not expecting Tony to be as thin and frail as he was, but as old friends do, they were soon chatting away and reminiscing, with Ernst being endlessly patient as Tony constantly repeated himself. They liked to sit out late in the afternoon with a glass of wine, a bowl of crisps and Ernst's small cigars. My role was to keep the wine and crisps topped up and just let them get on with it. I have some lovely photographs of the pair of them laughing and enjoying each other's company. They had carefully hidden the cigars from me in case I found out they were smoking, with apparently no idea I only had to glance out of the window to see them at it. The plumes of smoke gave them away.

Ernst was sad when he left, knowing this was probably the last time he would see Tony, although he was happy to have spent a pleasant time with him. Fortunately, I have not yet reached the age when old friends and contemporaries are dying, but it must be hard to see them falling away. Enclosed in the dementia bubble with Tony, it was easy for me to forget how his illness affected other people and it was useful to be reminded that, no matter how difficult or problematic it might be to arrange, other people did want to see Tony.

Earlier in the year, we'd had a contingent of Blairs to visit. Leo, Cherie, Nicky and Alex with baby Iris arrived and lots of photographs were taken with a proud but confused Tony. Apart from Cherie, he kept forgetting who everyone was, but as he liked babies he was content to sit on the sofa, cradling Iris while various members of his family posed with him. It was particularly difficult for Tony as he thought of Nicky as a young boy and couldn't equate this tall, bearded young chap with the person he remembered. The idea that Nicky was Iris's father was completely beyond Tony's comprehension, but nevertheless everyone enjoyed the visit and Tony was even more pleased when we all went out for lunch as he could, at least, understand what that was about. The contribution of other people including his family to the strategy of keeping Tony active was invaluable. I know most of the time he had no idea what was going on and things were explained to him that he immediately forgot, but no one in the family accepted dementia as any excuse to hide him away or exclude him from things. The focus was always on normalisation.

There were simple things I did to help Tony stay alert and engaged, such as taking the long route to where we were going when we went out in the car. This often meant driving through the hills and moors around where we live. He loved seeing the different moods and seasons of the countryside, and would always remark on how lucky we were to live in such a beautiful part of the world. Another strategy was to take him out with friends, or to visit them, so he was still socialising. On the whole, this worked well, but he could be quick to take offence if he thought someone was patronising him. A tone of voice might irritate him and he could occasionally fall into his old habit of verbally lashing out, though by now this was thankfully a rare occurrence. I think, in the end, he found being with other people too much work and he just wanted to be with me.

That was the case with holidays too. Previously, we had sometimes gone away with friends, particularly Brian and Betty whom we had known for a long time, but eventually we reached the point where Tony's behaviour made things too difficult. There was a time in Austria when he really upset Brian, and despite my urging Brian not to be offended, he was. It was easier for me as I had had years of practice in ignoring how dementia could make Tony unpleasant. When he was tired and physically not coping, this could result in verbal aggression; his almost constant repetition and confusion took some handling; his loss of inhibition, such as wandering around without his clothes or only partially dressed, could be startling. One of the most difficult things for friends to cope with was just how quickly he could forget them, even though they might have been having a conversation only moments earlier. Then, it was as if his memory had drained from him, which in all likelihood it had. So, when we went to Suffolk in March 2017 for what would turn out to be our last holiday, it was just the two of us.

Suffolk was a county we had always planned to visit, but hadn't got round to. I found a small, quiet cottage tucked away on an estate where we could take the dogs with us. Suffolk is a long way from where we live; I think it is possibly a long way from anywhere. We had to make frequent stops, but it was a successful journey, with Tony sleeping a lot of the time. When Tony was not sleeping, he liked to listen to music, which would quite often trigger memories for him. He would then tell me stories, most of which I had heard before, but I found this less irritating when I could focus on driving; and as long as I was lending him half an ear and asking the occasional question, he was satisfied. At least he was still talking to me, which was important. It helped to keep us connected.

Although Tony initially seemed fine after our journey, it had taken its toll on him. It was also clear he no longer wanted to be in a strange place with strange routines, even if

I was with him. I thought about abandoning the holiday and going straight home, but I then thought about undertaking the return journey so soon after we had arrived. I couldn't face it yet; I was tired too and knew I would struggle to cope if I tried. So, I cajoled and soothed him and got stroppy when I was tired of that. He might be ill, but I was not his paid nurse, we were a married couple, and sometimes a strop was the only answer, not just his prerogative; these things still had to work both ways sometimes.

We did work it out and things were fine in the end. I would drive to a beach, Walberswick being my favourite, park the car where Tony could look out at the sea and the big skies, and then I would walk the dogs – after first making sure Tony was well wrapped up in fleece blankets. I took lots of photographs, so he could see where I had been and vicariously enjoy the experience. After years of searching – and on a beach which must have thousands, if not millions of pebbles on it – I finally found two small pebbles that had holes all the way through. As we all know, those are the lucky ones. Back at the car, I showed them to Tony, who put them in his pocket to look after them for me. He understood their significance: that the search was over and the lucky pebbles were found.

Back home, Tony became needier than ever. It was no longer simply a question of knowing where I was at night, that I was in bed next to him should he need me, but having to know where I was at every moment. This was an exhausting new phase. If I was out in the garden and even if he could see me, he would stand at the front door watching; and I knew he was willing me to come back indoors. There was no compromise to this situation. Either I was outside doing what I wanted to do in the garden, or I was inside where he wanted me to be. The concept of my coming indoors after ten or twenty minutes was beyond him. Time meant nothing anymore. I might as well have said I was going back inside in two, three or four hours' time.

I found this really hard, this removal of my most basic autonomy, of my right to some choice, in order to calm his anxiety. Sometimes, I would just ignore him and he would then shout to me, asking if I wanted some tea. This was a quite a clever change of tactics to try to get me indoors, as we both knew he couldn't manage that task himself. In this respect, I had deliberately de-skilled him as he would flick the kettle on without first making sure there was water in it. Worried about the consequences, I had prevented him from doing it until he could no longer remember how to do it. I would also turn off the socket, which really floored him. He no longer made a mental connection between the kettle and the socket switch.

It is difficult to explain just how stressful it is, having someone following you around, needing your presence constantly – even if it is someone you love and care about. I had taken to banning Tony from the bathroom while I was having a shower just so I could have a few minutes' peace, but he soon came up with a master stroke. If he told me he needed to pee, he would have to go immediately and he would come banging and crashing into the bathroom, totally trashing any tranquillity I was hoping for. All those lotions and potions that offer soothing calm with just one squirt are as nothing when pitted against a man with dementia. His *coup de grâce* was flushing the toilet, which meant I'd be drenched with either boiling or freezing water. Twenty years of nagging him about toilet habits were now coming back to haunt me.

I recall one evening when I really had reached the end of my tether. Tony had driven me crazy all day with his mood swings, petulance and demands. I had to get away from him. I knew I couldn't leave him alone in the house, so I hid in the dark at the bottom of the cellar steps, secure in the knowledge that he would never think of looking for me there. I rested my head against the freezer and the steady thrum was comforting. All I wanted was the obliteration afforded by hours and hours of sleep – and I knew I was not going to get it. I could hear him moving about the house, calling for me, even enlisting the dogs in his search. Yet I didn't help him. I just sat there in the dark, listening. As he got closer, I knew I would have to reappear, so I took myself into the back yard and pretended I had been there all the time. When he found me his relief was palpable. Some part of me felt desperately sorry I had been so mean to him, while another part wanted to scream and scream at him to leave me alone.

How was I going to keep this up? How could I go on caring for him? The answer was, as it always had been: I didn't know. I would have to make it up as I went along and hope tomorrow would be a better day.

8.

The final days

Orkney in November is far from being the warmest place on the planet, but I was sweating. I had managed to cross the sea-soaked causeway to the Brough of Birsay without slipping over and was now toiling up the hill to the lighthouse. It wasn't raining; it was the kind of weather where the air is damp yet the brisk wind, which was making walking harder, did not blow the dampness away. I was only carrying a small rucksack, but it was heavy and I had to keep shoving my thumbs under the straps to try to ease the weight across my shoulders. Muttering and grumbling, I made my way past the lighthouse and out on to the cliffs, where the kind young woman in the Kirkwall Information Centre had told me the wind would be blowing in the right direction. I was relieved to get the rucksack off my back and stood there for a moment, getting my breath back and recovering from the slight dizziness brought on by carrying such a load. There was nobody there but me; out at sea, a single boat was travelling west to east. I assumed it was a fishing boat but couldn't really tell at that distance.

I sat down on a rock, opened my rucksack and pulled out the heavy plastic jar containing Tony's earthly remains. I hadn't realised just how heavy human ashes are. I had spent the last four days carrying him from home, along with the baggage I would need for ten days on Orkney. Not an easy task.

On arrival at Manchester airport, I'd explained to the woman at the check-in desk that I would need help going through security as I had my husband's ashes with me. As anticipated, the rucksack needed further inspection despite me and the staff member explaining it contained human ashes. When I went over to the security desk with my bag, the young woman there informed me that despite the cremation certificate and Tony's name on the jar, the jar itself would have to be opened. I kicked off loudly and uncompromisingly; with the check-in woman's support, it was agreed that all that was necessary was for security to swab around the lid. I watched whilst this was being done. And I watched as the four other security people, who were standing around whilst it was done, talked and laughed with each other. I broke down and sobbed. The complete lack of respect for Tony and for me was too much. I didn't have a tissue with me, but I was wearing a fleece and used the sleeve to mop my face and nose. It was the first time since Tony died that I had properly cried and it felt good to let go, even though I was in a busy public place.

I took him on board with me as hand luggage. I usually travel light, only taking a carry-on suitcase with the essentials, but I was beginning to find I was not quite as strong as I thought I was, as I struggled to get the rucksack in and out of the overhead locker. I did not tell the kind, young man who helped me why my bag was so heavy.

The person sitting next to me during the flight was an airline pilot. He was jolly and friendly, although at one point during our conversation he decided to explain to me the potential problems of propeller driven planes – one of the more serious being the propeller detaching and cutting through the cabin. Weirdly – my head was clearly in a very strange place at this time – the idea of falling to earth from a great height seemed vaguely attractive. No more thinking and no more grief. I didn't mention this to him as I didn't want him thinking I was a crazy woman, although I did tell him the story of an internal flight Tony and I had once endured in Jamaica. I'd been convinced the small plane was held together with Blu Tack and elastic bands, and that the only reason we landed safely in Montego Bay was by dint of the sheer force of my will power, holding the thing together.

The departure times didn't allow me to make a connecting flight to Kirkwall that day, so I spent the night in Aberdeen. I eventually made it to Smoogro and my rented bothy late the following afternoon. Tiny, isolated and right on the coast, the bothy suited my needs perfectly. I was finally alone with my thoughts and my pain, which was what I wanted and needed. I had stocked up on Warburtons thick white sliced bread and Twinings English breakfast tea, these having been my staple diet for the last few months – particularly as I had found being snuggled up in bed reading, with tea and toast to hand, was really comforting, as long as not too many crumbs made their way below the covers.

Of course, it was dark when I arrived at the bothy, but the lovely owner, Caroline, had supplied plenty of fuel for the wood burner, which I soon had blazing away. It was a good companion over the next two weeks. I'm sure there must have been a fire raiser at some point back in my Irish genetic history, as I never have a problem lighting a fire. I should have had a Brownie badge for it.

One of the best things that evening was opening the back door to see and hear the sea. There was just about enough moonlight to make out the white caps on the rollers as they hit the rocks. Although it was chilly, I opened a window slightly so I could lie in bed, watching the fire burn down and listening to the waves, and connecting my sad and sore spirit to the soothing elemental forces.

On the day the wind was blowing towards Norway, I set off with Tony for Birsay, but not having got my bearings properly, I went the wrong way. I had crossed the Churchill Barriers and reached St Margaret Hope before it occurred to me I might be wrong. I stopped at a village shop and was redirected north-west.

By now, I was in something of a tizz as I was worrying about how to deal with Tony's ashes. Exactly how do you cast them into the wind? I'm not squeamish, but I really didn't want to put my hand into the jar to scoop out handfuls of dust. Instead, I decided to walk to the cliff edge and shake the jar up and down, so Tony's ashes would be thrown into the wind. It turned out that I'd made the right choice as most of them were carried away on the breeze, with some settling on the cliff face.

Moving slightly back, I sat on a rock to talk to Tony. I had once tried to persuade him to go on holiday on Orkney, but he'd made it very clear there was no way he would ever visit a cold, windswept rock in the North Sea. I started to giggle at the thought that I had finally got my own way, but it wasn't simply that. Tony had always claimed he was a Viking and by releasing him into the wind blowing to Norway, I was returning him to his ancestral home, free to roam as he chose. Moreover, Birsay is itself an ancient Viking stronghold, so those ashes that didn't travel on the wind would be left with the remains of other ancient warriors.

It was certainly easier going back down the hill. I was able to amble, look around and chat to curious yet friendly sheep. At the bottom, I met a couple of women who were about to make their way up the slope. We stopped to chat and it was good to have what I hoped, from my side, was a friendly, normal kind of conversation. Looking back, I was still grappling with the idea of what 'normal' meant, particularly as my old normal was no longer my new normal, and I was still to create and get to grips with my new normal. There was a particular kind of madness to my grief that centred on the tension I felt between heartbreak and practicality. Facing that impenetrable wall of pain, both physical and emotional, the questions 'Do I have to?' and 'Should I go on?' circled on a loop in my brain – sometimes increasing in volume, sometimes sinking away to an insistent whisper. The answers were obvious, but provided no comfort.

I missed Tony so very much. All I wanted was to have him back again. I understood I was being selfish and that his dementia torment was now over. I even understood, as some people pointed out, that I knew his death was imminent – and in some ways this knowledge should have prepared me for it. Yet it didn't. I had lost Tony, the man I loved and married, as his dementia overwhelmed him. Truth be told, for some time I had been in a state of grief for what I had lost and was yet to lose, yet none of this prepared me for his final exit.

Tony died on Monday, 25 September 2017, at 10.40 p.m. His end was peaceful; he simply stopped breathing and his life was over. Cherie had arrived from London a couple of hours earlier and we sat on each side of the bed, holding his hands and singing to him, as we wanted him to know we were there. We played songs he loved such as Roberta Flack's 'The First Time Ever I Saw Your Face'. It was our song. And Bette

Midler's 'The Rose', which had always made Tony cry. He was terribly sentimental, so Cherie and I put our hearts and souls into it. We followed with 'Wind Beneath My Wings' and it was during this song that my Tony died. I don't know if this was corny or beautiful, but I do know that if he'd been able to, he would have looked straight at me, squeezed my hand and kissed me. I will never be able to find the words to explain just how much I loved him.

When Sophie, one of the district nurses who had been looking after Tony, arrived early the following morning, we had to get him ready to leave the house. We washed and dressed him, talking all the while so he would know what we were doing. It was the last kind thing I could ever do for him.

That night, once everyone had gone, I realised how very tired I was. How alone I was. What was I supposed to do now? I felt a physical pain but strangely not anywhere specific. I took some paracetamol to see if that would help and then I went to bed; but I couldn't sleep as my brain was still tuned into the nursery alarm I had set up to hear when Tony called out in the night. I had let the dogs come upstairs to sleep with me, the three of us huddled together, and each time I moved they would wake instantly, knowing something was wrong.

The following days passed in a blur; I was unable to think straight yet decisions still had to be made.

'How are you?' people asked as they took my hand or hugged me.

How many times do you have to answer what seem like the same questions? And, anyway, you've just forgotten what you've been asked. Sympathy in their eyes as they repeat the question more slowly and you close your eyes, so you don't have to see them.

Yet people's kindness and concern demanded a gracious response and I thanked them as they looked into my face – seeking what? Perhaps the truth. I was not fine. I was not coping. Please go away and fetch Tony back.

What did help was hearing the stories about Tony that so many people wanted to tell me. It was wonderful to know just how many lives he had touched with his kindness, humour and charm. Our friend Jean recently told me that years ago she hadn't known how to apply her make-up properly. I'm not quite sure how the issue had come up in their conversation, but Tony offered to show her how to do it. She turned him down, opting instead to try a House of Fraser make-up counter, but hadn't forgotten his kind, if somewhat unusual, offer.

But it was while I was out and about in Todmorden that I came to realise just how much he had become woven into the fabric of our small town. People who had sat next to him on the bus; chatted to him in the bookies; seen him recently in film and television repeats; older women who told me what a gentleman he was, always holding doors open for them; people who had stopped him on the streets because they recognised him and he had chatted to them; people from our tea shop and cafe haunts who knew Tony's order would always be fish pie and a pot of tea – and not to give him bread because he didn't want it as he had had to eat so much of it during the war.

There were obituaries in the national newspapers and on the television news bulletins, but it was the one in our local newspaper, the *Todmorden News*, which perfectly encapsulated all he was about. On the front page, they carried a photograph of us on the day I was made Mayor. Next to it was the headline: 'Star Actor, Political Campaigner and *Former Todmorden, Mayor's Consort* Tony Booth' – clearly the most important role that man ever played! Tony had an ego the size of a barn door, but he also had a softer, kinder side to his personality. I'm aware that some members of his family and those who knew him from his uproarious past would, quite reasonably, disagree with this description; but maybe I was the lucky one, who, despite some very tough times, also benefited from and enjoyed that gentler, more considerate Tony? It certainly helped to make our relationship last a long time. More than that, it gave me the strength to go on as Tony's health eventually collapsed. I had many good memories.

Only a few weeks before he died, Tony was sitting in the garden, smiling with pleasure, even though I had to wrap him in fleeces despite the warm day. His heart failure was taking its toll and he always felt cold. We were finding the days much easier than the nights, as Tony was beginning to suffer from hallucinations and he would also fall whenever he tried to get out of bed to go the bathroom. Although he was by now very thin, I was finding it more and more difficult to heave him off the floor and back on to the bed. His dementia meant that when I would ask and then shout at him to bend his knees to help me to get him off the floor, he didn't understand what I wanted.

Tony always seemed to fall between the end of the bed and a chest of drawers, the most narrow area in the bedroom. I have no idea how he managed to do that. I think he might have forgotten which way to turn for the bathroom. I would then struggle to drag him into a wider space, but this made the skin on his heels and lower back bleed with carpet burns. His feet were badly damaged when he was severely burned in an accident as a young man and nearly died. The sight of his blood and knowing my actions were causing the bleeding stressed me out as I tried to get him on to the chair next to the chest of drawers. Tony's distress would, almost inevitably, cause him to pee himself. He would then start shouting with humiliation. That left both of us shouting at each other.

Even if I managed to shove Tony on to the chair and then got his arm around my shoulders in an attempt to raise him to his feet, nine times out of ten he would fall off the chair. My goal was to throw the top half of him on to the bed and then haul his legs up behind him, struggling with the fact he wouldn't, or couldn't, bend his knees. Things were further complicated by the fact our bed was fairly high off the floor. It required weight-lifting skills – of which I had few. The whole experience was like going to hell in a handcart and took place almost every night.

One night, having tried and failed to get him off the floor, I just flipped and, after covering him with a duvet, decided to get back in bed and leave him where he was. I was so tired I almost fell asleep. It was the sound of Tony crying that stopped me. Leaping out of bed in a complete fury of exhaustion, I whipped the duvet off him, and, with the enraged strength of ten men, pulled him to his feet and managed to get him on the bed. Lying on the bed with a fresh set of bruises from his fall and the carpet burns still bleeding, he looked at me and said, 'I'm going to tell our Cherie you're beating me up.' I have no idea why I didn't just push him back on the floor, but instead I cleaned him up, changed his pyjamas and crawled into bed myself.

Deciding enough was enough, I spoke to Lydia, Tony's social worker, who was immediately on the case. She organised for a hospital bed to be delivered and for the district nurse to come out to assess Tony's needs. The bed was delivered almost immediately and was a godsend as it could be lowered. Our friends Henry and Kev were on hand to sort out the bedroom, dismantling our old bed and moving furniture ready for the hospital bed to go in. Poor Tony, who was by now only rarely out of bed, was parked on the couch in the room next door and wrapped up in a duvet, confused and anxious about what was happening.

By this stage, I could no longer trust my ability or strength to get him downstairs, so leaving him in bed was the safest option. I bought a nursery alarm, carrying my bit of it around the house with me, so I could hear him making any noise or movement. For me, a support network of people who understood our situation and who were willing to help out proved fundamental to my ability to care for Tony at home. Henry and Kev were part of that group and at the end of Tony's life I came to rely on their friendship and kindness.

Whilst hauling Tony off the floor was physically demanding, it was not as unnerving as his hallucinations. These began a few months before he died and the first one I can recall was when he woke me in the night to tell me, in a horrified whisper, there was a woman hiding under the table and she wanted to kill us both. Struggling to consciousness, it took me a few seconds to work out what he was saying.

'Don't be daft, there isn't a table in here! We're in bed,' I said.

'But she's there. I can see her,' he responded.

'Where?'

'There. Under the table at the end of the bed.'

'I'll put the lamp on and then you'll be able to see there's no one there.'

'Please don't do that – she'll be able to see us,' he begged, terrified. He seemed to be trapped in this frightening place, unable to budge from it, although he was talking and responding to me as I held him tight. 'Please don't let her get me,' he said, still whispering.

And so I lay there, holding this scared old man to me as close as I could, yet unable to pacify him. I leaned over and, switching on the lamp, said, 'Don't worry, I've got you.'

By now, he was almost screaming in panic and even when he could see there was no one there, his fear was such that it took him a few minutes to accept it. Once he was calm enough I got out of bed and turned all the lights on, as knowing he would need a pee at this point, I wanted to make sure he could see there was nothing and no one lurking about.

Peeing, whilst presenting a long-term issue, as it does for many older man, was even more urgent now. For a number of years, Tony had been worried about peeing himself, but now he was obsessional. Unfortunately, in his panic and concern, he frequently missed the toilet bowl as his focus was on not wetting himself, rather than on direction. When I was the Mayor I was often asked to visit care homes and one of the most difficult things about some of them was the smell of urine. I became fixated on trying to ensure that our house, particularly the bathroom, didn't smell. I must have kept sales of Dettol disinfectant particularly high in Todmorden, preferring the house to smell like a hospital rather than a urinal.

Once Tony was settled in a hospital bed, it quickly became clear that getting him to the bathroom was no longer an option. He also seemed to realise his bed was the safest place for him to be. He didn't move out of it for the three weeks before he died. I discussed options with the doctor and the district nurse and it was decided a Conveen sheath would be the answer. For the uninitiated, a Conveen is similar to a condom, with a tube attached at the end which feeds into a urine drainage bag. It's much less invasive than a catheter. Sarah, the district nurse, demonstrated how to use them – essentially, the same way as a condom. We stood, one on either side of the bed, looking at Tony, naked from the waist down. I understood my husband well enough to know that in his riotous heyday the thought of being starkers in front of two women would have had exactly the opposite effect to what was happening at this point.

Yet he continued to worry about peeing himself, no matter how many times he was told about the Conveen. It was one of the things that made him panic in the night. That and the bad dreams, which continued to haunt him even though a lamp was always left on in the room. It took me some while to work out that a dimmer switch on the overhead light was a better option than a lamp, as it creates less shadows.

It was not only Tony's physical comfort that I had to think about, but the needs of his family too, especially as he was now nearing the end of his life. He had a strained relationship with most of them, but by this point things were easier for him to cope with, as he couldn't recognise them and would simply chat and share stories with them. But did I have – should I have – enough generosity of spirit to let them know the seriousness of their dad's health and that it was time to say goodbye to him if they wanted to?

Over the years, I had watched from the sidelines as events, traumas and downright ill will had played out between them all. My primary concern was for Tony's wellbeing, but what was the right thing to do? In the end, I assigned myself the role of gatekeeper. I got in touch with his daughters, explaining the situation and saying we could make suitable arrangements should they wish to see him. That solution worked fine. He had visitors almost every day, with family and friends coming to see him. I don't know how, but he was still able to turn on the charm and chatter; and so, on one or two occasions, it was a little difficult to get people to understand that he was, in fact, tired and they needed to go. I don't think I was too rude as I herded them out of his bedroom. On the whole, I believe I made the right decisions.

But there were some things I could not control, including the fact that Tony was no longer eating. All he would consume was lemon-and-lime-flavoured water. It was a horrifying situation, as I was convinced he was slowly starving to death and all I could do was watch. He had been prescribed some sort of protein drink, but he hated the drinks and wouldn't co-operate by drinking them. Every now and then, he would announce he was hungry, but in reality he didn't want anything to eat: it was just something to say. What was really strange, given his overall deterioration and lack of sustenance, was that the carpet burns on his back began to heal. As always, he continued to defy expectation.

When the end came, it was rapid. Despite being told by the medical team it was only a matter of time before Tony died, a part of me thought he would probably go on for ever, as he didn't appear to be ready to give up. But in the space of a few days he descended into semi-consciousness and hallucinations. The next twenty-four hours were to be my greatest test of both love and stamina.

Whatever was in his head, it would not allow him any peace and just when I thought I had managed to calm him, he would start calling out again. Even when he did drift off into some kind of sleeping state, it was not an easy or restful space. I could not get into bed with him to give him physical reassurance, as hospital beds are much too narrow, so I sat in the room with him, hoping he would know I was there.

Whenever I did try to leave him to go and lie down for a while, he would soon be calling out for me. 'Steph, Steph, I'm so sorry,' he would repeat over and over, in a real state of distress. I had no idea what he was sorry for, and, whilst stroking his face, I would repeat over and over that I was OK.

It was one of the longest nights of my life, but fortunately the district nurse arrived early on the Monday morning. It was time to use Tony's end-of-life medication. I was numb with exhaustion and distress. How could this finally be happening? It was something to be talked about and prepared for, but never to face as a reality.

Once Tony had been given an injection, he descended into a calm space of unconsciousness, which I was grateful for, although he never spoke to me again. A few hours later, after the doctor had called, a syringe pump was set up for Tony and he then progressed peacefully, over the next few hours, to his death.

I did not know what to do with myself. I was in a state of suspended animation, waiting. Waiting for Cherie to arrive; I had promised I would call her, so she could be with her dad at the end. Waiting for the priest to arrive to give Tony the last rites. Waiting for Tony to die. Waiting, waiting, waiting. Trying to figure out how to breathe around the rock that had formed in my chest at some point during the day. Would the nausea I was feeling allow me to have tea and toast? Should I even be thinking about such things at a time like this? Please don't let me start crying. After all Tony and I have been through together, please let me hold it together until the very end.

I sat by his bed and talked to him. I knew he had been concerned about what would happen to me after he died. He was concerned about how I would cope without him to look after me. Remembering this and wanting to put his mind at rest, I whispered reassurances in his ear: 'It's fine. I will be fine. Please don't worry about me, you can go now. I love you. You can go.' Which, of course, was far from true. I did not want him to leave me, but I knew he had to. It is true, one of the toughest gifts of love is to let someone go. Sometimes it is too hard being a grown-up. As I sat at his side, I chatted about other things, reminding him of the good times we'd had and the places we had been together, until finally Cherie arrived and I was no longer alone.

I had not realised how bureaucratic death is. How literally, in a heartbeat, you go from being a wife to being a widow and how much form filling that entails. Then there is the funeral to arrange and, as for any other major life event, there are people, mainly relatives, who want to have their say about how it will be done.

The person I relied on most for the funeral was Peter, the funeral director from Warburtons. Todmorden is a small town, so Peter and I already knew each other, mainly from the cricket club. I was surprised by how many people told me they thought Tony's funeral would be in Liverpool, but we lived in Todmorden and his funeral was always going to be at our local Catholic church, St Joseph's. On the day, the church was packed. It was wonderful to see and I know Tony would have been delighted, too. The service was a traditional Catholic mass with the readings and hymns Tony had chosen. Todmorden Orchestra provided a string quartet to play Tony into the church and we processed behind him to the strains of the 'Londonderry Air'. There was only one moment when I wobbled, but Tony's son-in-law, Tony Blair, was walking beside me and instantly steadied me with a hand in the middle of my back. It was small, thoughtful gestures such as this that helped me get through the day.

One of the many things Tony taught me was public speaking, and at the crematorium I read W.H. Auden's 'Funeral Blues' for him:

> He was my North, my South, my East and West,
> My working week and my Sunday rest,
> My noon, my midnight, my talk, my song;
> I thought that love would last for ever: I was wrong.

This particular verse made me gasp for breath as my throat constricted with tears. I looked up to see other people crying, but I made it to the end. It was my personal farewell, on the day of his funeral, to my husband. In a public ceremony, it was our private moment; as was my decision to have Roberta Flack's 'The First Time Ever I Saw Your Face' as the final piece of music. Not as sophisticated as some of Tony's family might have liked, but our song, my choice.

And then the funeral was over and there was the rest of my life to get on with. The garden needed its autumn tidying, but

I didn't want to do it. This book needed writing, but I didn't want to do that either. I didn't know what to do – and I didn't know how to do it. I must have taken the dogs for walks. I must have gone shopping and read the papers and watched television, but I can't recollect anything. Getting through each day was a small triumph and then I got ill. Gastric flu, a kidney infection, a heavy cold followed by another kidney infection. I spent a lot of time snuggled up in bed or on the couch with Tony's dressing gown, which still had his smell on it. Pushing my face into it, I would close my eyes and pretend. Reality was too much.

I tried to follow the advice given by a number of people that I should accept invitations to do things, take part in activities, but being sociable requires strength, energy and a willingness I struggled to find. I know now this was all a normal part of grieving, including the health issues, but at the time I thought I was going mad. My head would not work properly. I needed antibiotics for the various infections and whilst I was at the surgery I asked my doctor if I should now come off citalopram, the antidepressant I was still taking. At the time it seemed like a reasonable question; after all, did I need them anymore, given that Tony had died? No, was the short answer, it would be too much for me to cope with. I was advised to come back in six months' time to discuss it then. Thank goodness I heeded her advice. Whilst the drugs had been a useful prop, one I could not have managed without,

I had no idea how hard it would be to come off them. The physical side effects were pretty unpleasant, with a lot of non-specific pain, but it was the crippling headaches that drove me to bed with strong painkillers – even though I was following a programme of gradual reduction. There were a few moments when I seriously considered not giving them up, such was the difficulty, but I did persist and I no longer take, and will hopefully never again need, antidepressants.

My life is improving as I regain physical and emotional strength, realising that giving up is not the answer, nor the one Tony would have wanted me to choose. The twenty-fifth of each month is still a marker of how many months it is since Tony died, especially during the first year. It is the special occasions that are particularly tough – wedding, birthday, Christmas – as you cope with the brutal knowledge that this time last year the person you loved was still alive. A week after Tony died, it would have been our wedding anniversary and the following week, his birthday. That was a bruising time, although to be honest we both usually forgot about our wedding anniversary. My friend Chris suggested Tony would have wanted to give me a piece of jewellery for our wedding anniversary, had he remembered. An unusual turquoise necklace from Element, Tony's favourite shop, was my choice. He bought me so many beautiful pieces from there, I could probably help to restock their shop in a crisis.

*

I was in Manchester before Christmas, buying presents. The weather was bitterly cold and I was shocked by how many young people were living on the streets, huddled in whatever they possessed, trying to keep warm from the freezing wind. Their pinched, grey faces were a testimony to our brutal and indifferent age. I was ashamed. Ashamed for lots of reasons, but particularly because I knew there were wardrobes and drawers full of Tony's warm clothing at home. Clothing that I had not known what to do with for the last few months and about which I, in my grief, couldn't bring myself to make decisions. I went home and filled bin bags with everything, all Tony's clothes, but I did find myself tearful as I looked at his shoes. Who could ever fill them? However, talking firmly to myself, they also went into a bag. I looked online for an emergency night shelter, the nearest one being in Rochdale. It was important to me the clothes went directly to the people who needed them and not to a charity shop. While those shops have an important function, they're still about making money, which inevitably makes them beyond the reach of the homeless. I loaded up the car with the bags and took them to the shelter. I kept Tony's dressing gown, which I now use as my snuggler and comforter, especially on those cold, long nights when I'm missing him the most.

Though his physical presence has gone, Tony is still very much alive in my heart and in my head, where we still carry on conversations. He would have given his approval to my decision – his only caveat, voiced in his own inimitable use of Anglo-Saxon, would have been to demand why it took me so long to figure it out.

Conclusion

I remember being seated next to Michael Foot years ago at a *Tribune* dinner. We chatted about various things before he suddenly asked me, 'What is it like, living with this rogue?' and pointed at Tony. I replied I had never been in so much trouble in my life and, starting to laugh, he said he could absolutely believe it. That was my life with Tony Booth and I can honestly say it was never boring. We undoubtedly weathered some tough and testing times, but boredom was never a problem. I have so much to look back on. Dancing in puddles during an impromptu street party in Arques in Languedoc; the look of astonishment on Tony's face when confronted by an angry waitress in New York; his insistence when we found two baby ducklings on Rievaulx Terrace in North Yorkshire that I should put them in my pocket and transport them to safety; when his heart was too frail for him to walk far, I would make the beachcombing expeditions alone, bringing back treasures to show him; the notes of encouragement I would find in my bag when I was about to speak publicly and he knew I was nervous. I still have all of these memories and many, many more; and they are what I hold on to as I work at – and still sometimes struggle to achieve – my new normal.

Caring for someone with dementia can at times be a strange and lonely world. Coming out of that space can be strange and lonely too. I have now managed to control some of my more unusual acquired habits. Such as repeating myself several times during the course of a conversation, something I did automatically with Tony until I was sure he understood what I was saying. It just makes me look and sound a little sad and weird now.

However, writing this book has given my life focus. In some ways, looking back over our history as I write has been cathartic, while in others it has been incredibly painful and I have found myself crying over the keyboard. I'm not sure how good tears and a runny nose are for a keyboard, but I think I've made a decent job of cleaning mine. After all, I still have a cupboard full of Dettol and associated products. Nowadays, I really can't make any more excuses about not thinking about the rest of my life and what I want to do with it. Tony was such a large presence in my life for such a long time, it's a big gap to fill.

But, whatever I decide to do next, one thing I am certain of is that I want to make good use of my experience of caring for Tony – and I know he would want that too. It is possible to care for someone with dementia at home, but why do government policy and bureaucratic systems make it so difficult? I know I've said it a dozen times before, but Alzheimer's is a wicked disease not only for the person who is suffering from it, but for everyone around them. David Baddiel, the comedian, novelist and television presenter, recently wrote an article about his father who has dementia. I was particularly struck by one of his comments: 'Memory, after all, is where we store our personality ... and dementia, surely, is the most terrible, the most complete hacker.' Coping with this truth, losing the person you love and then finding that the struggle for support, advice and benefits can be overwhelming makes for an unacceptably high personal price for any carer to pay. The organisation Carers UK estimates that unpaid care for someone with dementia is worth an estimated £11.6 billion a year to the economy – an extraordinary imbalance in commitment.

In December 2013, the G8 Health Ministers met in London to discuss how to shape an effective response to dementia. One of the outcomes of this meeting was the commitment to 'identify a cure or a disease-modifying therapy for dementia by 2025'. If the research industry can make good on this promise, that would be fantastic for dementia sufferers, post-2025. But, right now, that's only a pipe dream and there are thousands of people living every day with the reality of this disease. They can't wait for the promised 'jam tomorrow'. Statistics published by the Alzheimer's Society show that 80,000 people in this country are living with Alzheimer's – and these are only the ones we know about. Many people go undiagnosed. That figure of 80,000 is projected to pass a million by 2021. Each one of those numbers is a human being.

There is an All-Party Parliamentary Group on Dementia (APPG), a cross-party group made up of MPs and peers with an interest in dementia. Yet this is not good enough. In early 2018, I was talking to Norman Lamb MP, who is well respected for his knowledge and expertise in health issues, particularly mental health. Norman and I agreed the APPG needs to be more than a group of interested individuals. Its numbers should include scientific and health professionals as well as representatives from the vast pool of dementia carers in this country. None of us can wait until 2025. We need to start with innovative and sustainable policies that would quickly make a positive difference to the lives of people currently living with dementia. With all my new free time, I would put myself forward to be a member of such a committee. Like so many other experienced home carers, I've got much I need to talk about and be involved in.

But until I receive that call I intend to spend time catching up with family and friends. I'm looking forward to making quilts with Maggie. I'm going to start wading through and enjoying the pile of books I accumulated while Tony was ill. I will deal with neglected corners of my garden and am seriously pondering whether to get a couple of chickens. (Many years ago, Tony and I kept chickens until some idiot boy let his dog loose in our garden. I am still haunted by the sight of all those mutilated little corpses.) I will catch up on films I have missed. I'm only in my early sixties and I need to re-engage with a world that was gradually obscured to me by the demands of living in the dementia bubble.

I hope I'm sounding positive, because I know that whatever happens in the future, there will always be a part of me that just wants Tony back. . As I mentioned, the sound of his voice is still in my head and I have been caught out more than once by hearing his voice on the television. That is unnerving. When I think of him, the image I have is of the man I married before Alzheimer's claimed him. That is how I plan to remember him and the quite extraordinary life and love we shared. I will always miss you, Tony Booth.

Epilogue

Eulogy by Tony Blair

Tony was born on 9 October 1931, son of Vera and George, brother of Audrey and Bob, father of Cherie, Lyndsey, Jenia, Bronwen, Lauren, Emma, Lucy and Jo, whose mothers were Gale, Julie, Susie, Annabelle and Nancy, married also to Pat Phoenix and for the last nineteen years married to Steph, who was by his side as he passed away days before his eighty-sixth birthday.

But no mere details of biography could ever explain, constrain or contain the outsize, extraordinary, colourful, irrepressible character of the man whose life we celebrate today.

There are people about whom it is hard to say a lot, and people about whom it is impossible to say a little. Tony was definitely of the latter sort.

I certainly never met anyone like him, which at times I was thankful for! But in time, I came to know him, to like him and to admire him.

His upbringing shaped him. He was a star pupil at school, but when Tony was sixteen, his father – a merchant seaman –

fell down the hold of a ship, broke his pelvis, and since in those days there was no accident insurance for those injured at work, Tony had to leave school to be the family's breadwinner.

Shortly after, he did his national service. He became friendly with the colonel and perhaps more accurately the colonel's wife, who introduced him to a love of theatre and possibly other things; and his vocation in life was settled.

He was a natural: good looking, with presence, personality and verve. He was always going to succeed and before long he did.

He was part of that whole exploding Liverpool scene, which encompassed not just the Beatles of course, but Gerry and the Pacemakers, Cilla Black, Roger McGough, the Liverpool poets and many more.

It's impossible for this generation to get the enormity of the first real TV soap, *Till Death Us Do Part*. It was the most popular show in Britain in the days when everyone watched only BBC or ITV. It made Tony a household name.

Unfortunately fame also led him to a downward spiral of alcoholism, which limited his ambition at the very moment he should have fulfilled it, even though he still did remarkably well, appearing in films with, amongst others, John Wayne and Michael Caine.

The fire which nearly ended his life in 1979 turned out to be the saving of it. He reformed, giving up the booze and crazy lifestyle.

He showed in later life; he was a brilliant stage actor, with sublime gifts of timing and expression.

By then, he had entered my life.

He was an unusual father-in-law. One of the first times I met him, when I was just beginning as a barrister, he came round to see me at home and casually asked if I wanted to smoke a joint. When I declined, he said he assumed it was OK if he did, and thought it very odd when I said actually no. So he said, 'All right then, let's have a cup of tea.' I made it. He told me it was disgusting. And then proceeded to give me a lesson on how to make a decent cup of tea, something I have never forgotten.

I was the only one of my friends who had a father-in-law who appeared naked in *Oh! Calcutta!* and starred in the *Confessions* films. And I loved that his mum, the wonderful Vera, who adored him, when she first heard of the films, believed it was probably something to do with religion and the priesthood.

People said he was always difficult with me politically, but he wasn't. In fact, given the provocations of New Labour to such a long-standing Labour activist like Tony, he was immensely restrained. More than that, he showed me a kindness and solidarity throughout my time as Prime Minister which I found of great comfort. The pot smoking, however, remained something of an issue. There was a time in Downing Street when I came up to the flat for a meeting with a senior civil servant and as we both wrinkled our noses, the civil servant said, 'If I didn't know any better I would think you had been smoking weed, Prime Minister,' to which I laughed nervously. Mind you, Tony always reminded me that he had been in Downing Street long before me, as indeed he had been, in Harold Wilson's time.

His politics were unashamedly on the Left, but from that progressive side of politics which embraced social liberalism and a fierce defence of human freedom.

He was always a rebel. Never a conformist. Any cause he espoused, he fought full on. When he perceived the actors' union Equity was being led in a conservative direction he didn't like, he took on the entire establishment of his own profession and was elected as Union President when no one thought he had a chance.

He was huge fun, full of stories, a passionate Liverpool football fan, and with a charm that was legendary.

Actor, rebel, raconteur, and in his final years much to his pleasure: Consort to the Lady Mayor of Todmorden and proud inhabitant of this beautiful town. He found genuine happiness here, felt completely at home and on behalf of all the family I would like to thank the people of Todmorden for the affection you gave him. It meant so much to him and to Steph.

Steph looked after Tony, tended him with love and care, especially through the difficulty of Alzheimer's and I know he lived as long as he did and with the joy he experienced in his old age as a result of Steph and her love for him.

Thanks to Steph, Tony died at home as he wished.

Shortly before he died, he saw his grandson Euan and from his deep love of Shakespeare, which remained with him to the end, he quoted the words of Polonius: 'This above all: to thine own self be true.'

It is a fitting epitaph for Tony. Nothing about him was ordinary. Not much was conventional. A lot was controversial. But everything he did he did to the full. Career, relationships, family, work, everything from causes to conversations, he did it and said it as he thought it.

To his own self, he was true. And that is why, despite it all, we loved him and will miss him deeply.

Things I wish
I'd known

My garden remains my place for reflection, where I can think through things while plotting the autumnal reshaping of the flower beds. One of the things to have preoccupied my thoughts since Tony died is what advice I would give to people who find themselves caring for someone with dementia. Things I wish I had known or been told when Tony was first diagnosed. I've put together a few ideas I hope might be helpful – and that is all they are, my thoughts gleaned from my experience.

- Dementia is a difficult disease to diagnose. We can all be forgetful: how many times have you got to the top of the stairs and completely forgotten why you are there? This is not dementia. Signs of confusion are the clearest indicators that perhaps something more serious is going on. For example, I became concerned when I realised Tony was beginning to mix up reality with the fictional characters in the book he was reading. Talk to your GP if you notice any significant signs of confusion in your loved one.

- Do not allow yourself to be shunted out of the doctor's office with the blithe assumption you will be able to cope. That wouldn't happen with any other long-term disease and it shouldn't happen with dementia. Dementia is unique to the person who has it, meaning care and support have to be specific to their needs. Do not worry about being assertive. You are the carer and you know them best, no matter what the doctor or other people are telling you.

- While you're getting organised, it's also a good time to sort out your finances. I didn't find the Department for Work and Pensions (DWP) to be the most helpful of organisations and you will need to push hard to find out about the benefits and allowances you may be entitled to. Don't give up on this. I did and then too late found I was probably entitled to a Carer's Allowance.

- Sort out legal matters early, including making wills and organising power of attorney. Don't wait for a crisis or, worse, get to the point when the person with dementia is no longer able to give informed consent. Power of attorney will allow you to deal with important matters, including the health and benefits system on their behalf, as and when they are no longer able to do so.

- Make it a priority to find a good care home – one where you would be happy to leave them, so you can have a guilt-free, or at least a less guilty, respite break. They are out there, so arrange to visit. Don't be afraid to ask questions and keep looking until you find one that is suitable for your needs. This took me too long to learn and I didn't do Tony or myself any favours by delaying it.

- Don't be like me and wait until you hit breaking point before contacting social services. They can offer different kinds of support, including day centres. Tony started going to a centre through a social services referral and it was a massive help in terms of having time and space to myself.

- The person with dementia can find it difficult to accept their illness, but it is sometimes the reactions of other people, particularly family members, that may be surprising and unhelpful. Even when the evidence is clear, some refuse to accept the diagnosis. I have certainly found this to be true. I realise now it would have been better for everyone if I had not allowed myself to become distressed by their lack of understanding and support. Not everyone reacts well in a crisis. A critical lesson to learn as a carer is to focus on the positive. Prioritise what is helpful and move on from what is not.

- For a short while after Tony was diagnosed, people we knew would cross the street to avoid us simply because they had no idea what to say. This can be really hurtful, but my advice would be not to worry about what other people are thinking, there is no shame in dementia. If they are finding it difficult, that's something they will need to overcome. I found, for the most part, that once people were over their initial fears, things went back to how they were.

- One of the most important points I want to get across is to try not to feel guilty. I struggled with that, we all struggle with it, but there will be good days, not so good days and then there will be truly awful days. On the awful days, when you feel your head might just explode, you are allowed to grumble or even to shout at your partner. You are a human being and you do not become a saint when you become a carer. With the best will in the world, it is hard to answer a repeated question as if it is the first time of asking or listen with rapt attention when you are being told the same story again and again.

- Don't panic. Don't assume it is all immediately downhill following the diagnosis. There may well be a good few years before things begin to get really difficult.

- Have fun together. Make a joint bucket list and then do as much of it as you can. You will need these memories to hold on to when the person you love starts to retreat from life and from you. Our trip to Languedoc was about ticking things off the list, but when Tony was too frail for that sort of journey, I joined the National Trust and the Royal Horticultural Society. Both organisations have pleasant gardens with a plentiful supply of benches for rest stops and they usually have a nice tea room. These were the perfect ingredients for Tony when we had a day out.

- We were lucky as we didn't have to travel to enjoy a garden. Even a small patch filled with scented flowers – such as roses and lavender – and butterfly-attracting plants like buddleia can provide a calm and restful space. Todmorden in Bloom run an annual gardening competition and this year (2018) I won Gold for our small garden. The garden I created for Tony. He would have been thrilled.

- Local groups can be a good source of support. I always avoided the ones specifically for carers as any free time I had was for me and I would seize that time to do things I wanted to do beyond the dementia bubble. I helped to set up Dementia Friendly Todmorden and know there is another excellent one in Rothwell near Leeds. Both these groups have cafes where the general public as well as those with dementia and their carers can come together. They have an important role not just in offering support and advice, but in normalising dementia.

- Face up to the fact that palliative end-of-life care must be discussed sooner rather than later. With everything else going on, this can be a really tough issue to tackle and finding the right moment is the first hurdle.

- Sometimes, it can feel like the easiest thing to do is to jump in and do things for them. But no matter how frustrating it is, try not to. A skill forgotten is a skill that can never be relearned. That said, I didn't always follow my own advice, particularly if I was in a hurry. Getting dressed used to take Tony for ever, but being able to do so meant he kept some independence and dignity. For some reason I don't understand I didn't want to have to dress him. It always felt that was a step too far in my caring for him. Buttons were the particular nightmare and long-sleeved T-shirts and fleece jackets were the solution. The zips on the jacket were a nuisance, but I didn't mind fastening those for him.

- Towards the end Tony slept a lot during the day, which often meant he was restless at night. He also became afraid of the dark, especially after he began suffering from hallucinations. I discovered a dimmer switch in the bedroom was more calming for him than a lamp left on. Perhaps because the dimmer created a more ambient light and didn't seem to create so many shadows. We were still sharing a bedroom and I found it also made it easier for me to sleep too. I only wish I had discovered this simple solution much sooner than I did.

- Our dogs were a comfort to Tony. Pets give unconditional love and affection, the kind of easy, undemanding relationship people with dementia need. You can always borrow a dog for a few hours if you think this would work for you – and then you have the added bonus of not having to look after them full-time!

- Red wine. I have been reliably informed it is full of antioxidants and they are brilliant for reducing stress levels. I'm not suggesting for one moment carers should become dependent on alcohol, but sometimes the sound of the cork being pulled from a bottle of wine can be one of the most wonderful and soothing sounds. Relax, put your feet up and enjoy a glass of wine. It might even qualify as one of your five a day....

There are organisations out there offering help and support, but here are just a few you might find helpful. Don't be afraid to cherry pick, taking only what is useful for your current situation. You can always go back to them as and when things change:

- **Age UK**: for advice and information on money, care or health, visit: ageuk.org.uk

- **Care Quality Commission (CQC)**: they inspect care homes and provide a good starting point when you are looking for respite care. For more information, visit: www.cqc.org.uk

- **Alzheimer's Society**: a care and research charity for people with dementia and their carers. Services include the National Dementia Helpline: tel. 0300 222 11 22. To learn more, visit: alzheimers.org.uk

- **Shared Lives Plus**: an alternative and flexible service provided by individuals and families in local communities. It is not yet a national organisation, but find out more by calling 0151 227 3499.

- **Social services**: in the UK, these can be accessed through your local council's Adult and Social Care service. They can help you to find out what benefits you might be entitled to and which support services are available in your area. Their contact details will be on the council website.

- **Admiral Nurses**: they provide specialist dementia support, working mostly in the community for the NHS, but also in care homes, hospices and hospitals. They work with people and families affected by all types of dementia and can be contacted through the Dementia UK Helpline: tel. 0800 888 6678.

Acknowledgements

I must first give grateful thanks to Conor Goodman, the Features Editor at the *Irish Times* who commissioned my 'Married to Alzheimer's' articles. He allowed me the freedom to write about whatever was on my mind at any given time. It is down to his belief that the articles were good enough to form the basis for a book that you are reading this now. My thanks must also go to Nira Begum, my editor at Penguin Random House, who has encouraged, supported and where necessary chivvied me.

Writing this book has not always been easy, but I have good friends who have kept me going with their love and thoughtfulness, both during the long months of Tony's illness and since his death. Thank you to Jean and John Adams, Chris Potter, Christine Perry, Karen Smith and John and Ollie Gibbons, Betty and Brian Colley, Ernst Walder, Kevin McDougall, Alex Powell, Maggie Pearson and Matthew Maisey. As the legendary Joe Cocker sang, 'I get by with a little help from my friends.'

A special thank-you to the lovely people of Todmorden, including Henry Damer who, through his perfectionist joinery, plumbing and other skills, adapted our house, making it possible for Tony to remain at home. Henry was endlessly patient with Tony, chatting away and listening for the umpteenth time to his stories. He was latterly joined by his mate Kev Heys, especially at the end of Tony's life when beds needed to be dismantled and furniture moved to accommodate Tony's medical needs. Thanks to Emma C. and Rick, whose advice proved crucial to my having the time and space to write. And to all those kind-hearted souls who have taken the time to give me hugs and ask how I am: those small gestures have meant more than I can say.

Finally, love and thanks to our families, mine and Tony's, who have always been and who remain a vital thread in the fabric of our lives.